T0283087

The Lessons

The Lessons

**How I Learned to Manage
My Mental Health and
How You Can Too**

Nile Wilson

Vermilion
LONDON

1

Vermilion, an imprint of Ebury Publishing
20 Vauxhall Bridge Road
London SW1V 2SA

Vermilion is part of the Penguin Random House group of companies whose
addresses can be found at global.penguinrandomhouse.com

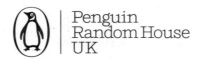

Penguin
Random House
UK

First published by Vermilion in 2024

www.penguin.co.uk

A CIP catalogue record for this book is available from the British Library

ISBN 9781785044809

Typeset in 11/18 pt ITC Galliard Std by Jouve (UK), Milton Keynes.
Printed and bound in Great Britain by Clays Ltd, Elcograf S.p.A.

The authorised representative in the EEA is Penguin Random House Ireland,
Morrison Chambers, 32 Nassau Street, Dublin D02 YH68

Penguin Random House is committed to a sustainable future
for our business, our readers and our planet. This book is made
from Forest Stewardship Council® certified paper.

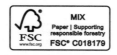

CONTENTS

WHY I WANT TO TALK TO YOU

Ey up!

For those of you who don't who I am, I'm Nile Wilson and I used to do roly-polies for a living!

Well, more accurately, I used to be an Olympic gymnast. I'm a lad from Leeds and, as I'm writing, I'm 28 years old. What's for sure is that my life has never been anything but colourful.

I made Olympic history at 20 years old by winning Team GB's first ever medal on the horizontal bar (or high bar, as it's sometimes called).

I have built a huge social-media following, with over 1.5 million subscribers on YouTube, and I was named as one of the top 50 influencers in the UK by the *Sunday Times*.

I am an owner of multiple businesses.

I have a penthouse apartment in Leeds.

I have an incredible family around me.

So, I guess I'm what a lot of people think is a 'success'.

Well . . . there is more for you to know about me.

I have struggled enormously with my mental health.

I have found myself crying in the middle of the night for no apparent reason while crippled with anxiety.

I have just finished a 12-month driving ban.

I have struggled with my gambling and drinking.

I have behaved in ways that I am not proud of and I've hurt people.

I need help all the time.

Yeah . . . so that's me. A contradiction in so many ways. From the outside, I look bulletproof, but on the inside there has been a different story going on. I have reached some incredible highs and crashed to some of the darkest lows where I have even contemplated suicide.

I think everybody, maybe even including myself, believes Olympians should have all the answers. We are the ones who have reached the peak of performance under the craziest pressure while the world watched us. We have been celebrated, adored and held up as the people everyone else should aspire to be. I know that I saw Olympians as superhumans when I was young, and when I reached that level I expected to feel that strong. But I definitely haven't always felt like that inside. The truth is that I have had far more questions about myself than answers to give anyone else. At times I have played up to that superhuman persona of an Olympian, while inside my head I have felt weak and suffocated. Alcohol and gambling helped me temporarily numb those feelings, but in the end they dragged me down even further.

Since I had to retire from elite gymnastics in 2019, it has felt like my life has taken every possible turn it could and, though I didn't necessarily realise it at the time, I have learned so much about who I am along the way. Some of those lessons were more than a little uncomfortable – I haven't always liked what I have found out about myself. It's true that I took many steps forward during this time, but maybe just as many back. Honestly, it has been fucking tough, but I have come through it and I'm incredibly proud about that. I feel like I have so much to share with you within this book.

So, why have I chosen *now* to write this book?

This was actually a really important question for me to answer in my head before I started writing this. I have always been honest and transparent about my challenges with my mental health, which have been a significant part of my life for the last three or four years. However, I believe there is a huge responsibility when it comes to sharing advice or experience in this area because it affects so many people's lives enormously. If I was going to step out in this way and share the lessons I've learned then I needed to be sure that I was in the right mental space to do so. Thankfully, I know that I am, but I need to explain that further. I know I am ready to write this book but it doesn't mean that I am in any way 'cured' of mental health issues. Far from it. I still have challenges. I'm not perfect and I am still capable of making mistakes. Just like anyone. That's the thing about mental health, you don't just wake up one day and go, 'I've solved it!' It's like any area of your health – you need to respect it enough to keep your eye on it all the time. When you neglect it, it comes back around to bite you.

So, I'm not sitting here, writing this, pretending to be someone who has cracked the puzzle as to how to never have poor mental health – it doesn't work like that. But, and it is a big 'but', the last 12 to 18 months have been truly transformational for me. I feel like I have turned a corner and started to understand the things that I have needed to. My mental health has improved dramatically during this time, and when things have happened that could have caused me to mentally fall off a cliff, I didn't. I have managed to find ways of not reacting unhealthily to stressful situations, which in the past would have set off a series of events creating a downward spiral in which I feel extreme anxiety and a dark depression. Finally, I feel like I am handling my mental health with knowledge and self-awareness, rather than as a person feeling their way through the dark.

It is for this reason that I know I'm ready to write this book and share with you all that I have learned during this time. I want to be a powerful young voice to help people with their mental health challenges. The strongest emotion

4

I have felt during my darkest times has been loneliness, and I don't want anyone to feel that – it's fucking horrible. We can be surrounded by people and yet feel desperately alone in our heads. I know that by speaking out, I can be a serious force in helping with these challenges, and this book is a reflection of that.

In 2022, I won one of ITV's flagship television shows *Dancing on Ice* in front of millions of people. It was a massive thing to happen to me for lots of reasons, and I'll explain why that was in a bit. But it nearly didn't happen at all. Not many people will know this, but when my agent got me an audition for the show, I was in a pretty bad place. *Dancing on Ice* was a huge opportunity and yet I almost blew it before I'd even turned up.

In early 2019, I suffered a neck injury while at a British Gymnastics training camp in Germany. I was practising my floor routine and as I did a tumble, I felt a sharp 'pop' in my neck. It was big enough for me not to be able to ignore it. Within hours, the pain was as bad as I have ever felt in my life. It was horrific. Ten out of ten pain. I would eventually find out that a disc in my neck was now pushing straight into a nerve. The injury was so bad that I needed surgery. In the end, it finished my career. I had thought I'd be able to return to gymnastics after the surgery, but every time I tried, my body broke down due to the toll the injury had taken on me.

When I realised it was all over, I started to feel completely lost. Not having the opportunity to perform in front of people left a huge void in my life. It had been such a passion for me – I had fallen in love with performing gymnastics aged four, and it truly felt part of who I was as a person. So when the opportunity to audition for *Dancing on Ice* came up, I knew that it would mean a chance for me to do that again in front of millions of people watching on television. It almost didn't matter that it was ice skating, a whole different sport – I was desperate for it. And yet at that time in my life, I still couldn't hold it together even to be on time for the audition.

I had just started serving that 12-month driving ban, my mental health was shot to pieces and I was making poor decisions around alcohol. I knew that my agent had fought for me to get that audition. But instead of being there bright and early, I turned up an hour and a half late for it. I bloody slept through my alarm, didn't I, and missed my train to Manchester. I had to jump in a cab as soon as I woke up. It was awful and embarrassing – but also a true reflection of where I was then in my life.

By some miracle, they liked me at the audition despite my lateness, and I got one of the last slots on the show. To this day, I look back on that and think how lucky I was. If I hadn't got on the show, would I have been able to get myself where I am today? Honestly . . . I don't know. Not only was I given the opportunity to perform again, but I was also given a structure again around training and preparing for the live shows. That structure was so important, giving me the routine, purpose and direction that I craved after retiring. Now I could be back to being an athlete, even if it was with ice skates on rather than flying around a metal bar. The whole experience all the way to the final proved to be truly incredible.

Yet, there was something that came out of *Dancing on Ice* that I didn't expect at all. Yes, I got the experience of being on TV in front of millions of people and the incredible accolade of ultimately winning the final. There's no question that I got a massive buzz off the fact that people were so excited about my performances that they voted for me to win. At the time, I thought this was the thing I'd been searching for since retiring from gymnastics. But when I came out the other end of it having achieved everything that I wanted, I realised, to my surprise, that I didn't actually need the validation of performing in front of all these people as much as I thought I did.

Now, don't get me wrong, I *loved* the whole experience and will be forever grateful to the show for the opportunity, but this realisation at the end of it was a huge breakthrough for me. I could enjoy striving for something but didn't desperately *need* it to define my happiness. Lifting the trophy in the final was magical, but what was far better was seeing my friends and family afterwards and us laughing, dancing and spending time together. I realised that I didn't need to keep searching and chasing for something – everything I needed was right there in front of me, and it was within my experience with the people surrounding me in my life. Suddenly I felt like I had more clarity and my eyes were open.

After other big events in my life, mainly gymnastics competitions, if I had performed brilliantly in them, like the Olympics final, then I would feel like I could fly. If it had all gone wrong, like in the European Games in 2015, which I'll tell you all about shortly, then my whole world would feel like it was falling apart. Yet, this time, I wasn't necessarily on top of the world or having an enormous crash – I was more level about it all. It was wonderful, with lifetime memories, but, maybe for the first time in my life, my achievement didn't have an enormous impact on my overall happiness. In the past, my results in gymnastics had a dangerous attachment to whether I would feel happy or not. I realised then that over the previous six months I had unknowingly begun to learn so much about myself and how to manage my mental health.

I hope there are things in this book that will help everyone. But one specific reason why I wanted to write it is that I still think men in particular struggle to talk openly about their mental health, and I completely understand that. Part of masculinity is wanting to be strong, a leader and a protector – and if you don't, it can be incredibly lonely and you feel like a failure. What I want to do is give people the courage to be able to just accept where they are at. This doesn't necessarily mean you have to shout out your pain to the world, but just for you to get to a place where you can speak to somebody and not feel guilty or ashamed about it. When you do that, you can feel less lonely, which gives you strength to face challenges.

If a person is feeling less-than because they don't feel like they are matching up to their own expectations then I want them to unlock that potential of being honest about it. Rather than see it as a weakness, I would love to help people understand that there is great power in it. Just because we're experiencing feelings of sadness and hopelessness, it doesn't mean that we can't still be a leader, a provider and a strong person. By talking about it, addressing the pain and under-standing it, we actually empower ourselves to be stronger people – whatever that looks like for each individual. I know that as a young man, I used to see showing vulnerability as being a weakness; now I see it as a great strength.

What follows from that is knowing more about who you are and then finding ways to be disciplined enough to do the things that you know are going to be good for you. This is actually a really important point – you can know what you need to do but then you need to action it. My self-awareness around this has increased massively. I've been talking about all of this for the last four years, but it is only in the last eighteen months that I've been brave enough to implement it and be more consistent with it.

One of the main ways this has manifested in my own life is around drinking. The truth is that I don't always like who I am when I have been drinking, and drinking tends to happen when I have got myself in a hole with my mental health – so, I don't want to get in that hole in the first place. I don't want to be that guy who struggles to have a conversation, stuck in his own head all day, every day and just hides away. I want my brain to be buzzing in a good way; I want to be able to have fun with my friends and family. The alternative is a crap version of Nile that's in pain and difficult to be around.

Just one of the important things I have learned is that when I get myself into a dark place with my mental health, I subconsciously don't want to get out of it. As back-to-front as that sounds, I would rather stay in the darkness because that is what I am used to. It's bad, but it's also weirdly comfortable. Maybe this is something you can relate to? Are there situations in your life that are not healthy but strangely you feel more at ease with that struggle than trying to find a solution? Internally, I think, 'I don't know how I've got here, but this is what it is.' And that's usually when I look for an escape with something like alcohol. They feed into each other and then all of a sudden, after two, three or four months, I realise, 'I'm really not good here.' But you just see it as being where you operate, and you just try to keep the wheels turning. I now know that I don't want that. That's not a good way to live.

My priority in life is not winning medals or trophies any-more; it is consistently doing the things that I know make me healthy and feel good. The lessons I have learned over the last few years have given me tools that have genuinely trans-formed my life. I am going to share all of these with you because I know how much they can do for your life as well. I feel incredibly excited for the opportunity that lies ahead for you! My lessons might be different to someone else's and you might find that you want to try to apply something I explain here in a different way. But they are real, they have changed so much for me and they can do the same for you.

I want you to read this book from start to finish because the order is important. Also, please have a notebook to hand so you can note down the things that hit home for you as we go through each topic. I am going to continually ask you to self-reflect, and writing down your thoughts will help you enormously with that.

We are going to look at various aspects of self-awareness so that you can understand yourself better. The relationship we have with ourselves is the most important one we can have, and this is one of the main things I want to help you with. I am also going to give you practical advice that you can put into action on a daily basis – because managing our mental health is an ongoing, everyday process. Most importantly, I am not going to put you under pressure or place you in a position where you are comparing yourself with others. I am definitely not a 'box-ticking' guy who is just going to set you things to do as part of a generalised list. My advice is as much about helping you find what works for you as anything. I even think some of my advice might shock you!

Ultimately, I want you to be the best version of you, whatever that feels like – and it gives me a buzz just to tell you that. The darkness cripples our creativity, our conversations, our curiosity, our laugher and who we are meant to be. We are going to have days when we don't feel OK, and that's OK. There is no such thing as perfect and trying to chase it will lead us off down a dead end. That doesn't mean that we shouldn't try to achieve wonderful things, but if that involves a search for perfection in some way, whether in a relationship, job or something else, it can suffocate our happiness. This is about being able to ride the ups and downs of life. When we are being the best we can be, everything flows so much more easily. We can reach our goals, however ambitious they are, and most importantly, we are happy and healthy.

As a young lad from Leeds, I genuinely feel privileged and humbled to be able to share this book with you.

Let's do this!

THE FALL

I want to start this book with a chapter that brings us all together to recognise what that fall into the deep hole of poor mental health feels like. I know that the first time I suffered from anxiety and depression, I thought I was the only person in the world who felt like that. You might be reading this feeling the same? Maybe you feel or have felt that no one understands the struggle you have with your mental health? That loneliness is a significant part of the desperate and dark feelings that we experience. This chapter is aimed at tackling this by putting into words how we feel during these times so that we can recognise that we are not alone with it.

Here are some words that I think of when I contemplate that hole: suffocating, out of control, breathless, crippling, head-fuck, alone, darkness upon darkness, fucking horrible.

All of these are exactly why poor mental health can be so

debilitating for someone. But what is often forgotten is that you don't suddenly feel all these things. Most of us don't feel fantastic one day and then wake up the next day feeling like our world has caved in. It's not like going from a hundred to zero in a flash – this thing is damn sneaky. It creeps up on you. And at the very start of a downward spiral you don't necessarily recognise the path you're about to go on – it is too subtle for that. That is why you can suddenly look around and find yourself in a challenging place mentally, then wonder how you ever got there. And why it is so hard for people around you to understand.

If I could put that downward spiral into words, it would go something like this.

'I'm good.'

'I'm pretty good.'

'I'm fine.'

'I'm fine.'

'I'm fine.'

'OK, I'm not fine but it's fine.'

'It's fine.'

'I'm fucked.'

My use of the word 'fine' has always been very telling. It's a nothing word really. A stopgap. I use it when all is not well but I won't admit it to myself, so 'fine' gives me a get-out. It's also a reflection of how the decline is gradual – 'fine' is that middle territory from good to shit that you can live in for quite a while without thinking much about it. Only when you have started to recover can you track back to where it all began. This slow slide has caught me out a lot, and it is why I now maintain a healthy respect for what can happen and the need for me to see the signs early. If ever I take my eye off my mental health and what keeps me healthy or, even worse, think I'm 'cured', I find myself sliding back to that place again without even realising that the process has started.

Sometimes there is an obvious trigger for this spiral, and at other times, there won't be. This is a really important point to remember. There doesn't have to be something that's clearly gone wrong in your life to make you feel like something is very wrong. This can often be a really confusing part of experiencing poor mental health. It feels like there should be a reason for it but there isn't always an obvious one to be found. However, what I have learned over time is that when I have fallen into a downward spiral, it has been a compounding of decisions, a chain of events and a series of feelings that all seem individually small but add up over time until they feel like a huge monster or a mountain. The best analogy I can give to explain this is a bathtub gradually filling up with water. The bath is never overflowing until it *is* overflowing. There isn't an actual problem until that one extra drop of water causes it to overflow. There may have been times to get concerned while the bath water was approaching the top, but until that last extra drop lands, you might have felt like you didn't need to do anything. That is exactly the same process I am talking about with mental health. Both you and the people around you might not necessarily see the problem that is coming until that one extra thing pushes you over the edge. To continue this analogy, our bath also overflows when we have forgotten to check on it, when we have taken our eye off it. Mental health is exactly like that. When we don't pay attention to it or respect it enough, then we can all of a sudden have a problem.

If you're not sure what a downward spiral might look like – or if you know only too well but feel like you are alone in the dark pit you have slid into – let me tell you about one of my worst. As I mentioned before, I suffered a neck injury in 2019, while away at a Great Britain training camp in Germany. The pain was horrific and the journey home on the plane was terrible. Every bump or movement caused a jolt of pain through my neck. I wanted to be home more than anything. However, even when I got home it was still bad. There was a two-week wait for surgery and it was the most excruciating fortnight of my life. And it wasn't just about the physical pain. The timing and nature of this injury was really significant for me in my bid to take part in the Tokyo 2020 Olympics – I was now facing a major problem. The physical pain was obvious, but the mental pain was an intense internal worry about the future and whether I would recover in time for the Olympics, or ever, for that matter. An injury to your neck makes you feel vulnerable in so many ways because it's such a pivotal part of the human body and the movements we can make. When I had such pain in it, I felt physically vulnerable, even defenceless. All of this added to the mental agony I felt.

I couldn't handle the pain. I just wanted out from it. So, to escape, I drank a lot of alcohol and took a lot of painkillers during my wait for surgery. At this point, you might be thinking that wasn't *so* bad because, well, whatever gets you through and recovery couldn't start until after surgery anyway. But it doesn't work like that for me. I had already begun a process of mentally trying to escape the situation. Drugs and alcohol were my way of doing this. This meant that when I came out of surgery, the same anxiousness – general and about the future – was still haunting me. I still couldn't train so I lacked purpose, was restless and bored. And guess what? I still didn't want to sit with it, I still didn't want to deal with it. The understandable but not necessarily helpful dynamic in this sort of situation is that lots of people have sympathy for you so you get away with a lot of things. Being withdrawn or sad, or drinking a lot are things that people might expect during this time, so they don't necessarily notice that it might be the start of a major problem.

Over the following weeks and months, I started to dismantle almost every healthy structure I had. It's the strangest thing to describe because it doesn't make any sense. Just when I most needed healthy people and habits around me, the slide that I was on became a self-perpetuating cycle. I felt rubbish so I isolated and drank more alcohol, which in turn made me feel more rubbish, and then I repeated it all. It made no sense, especially to my family and friends, but it's the vicious cycle that I found myself in.

As I pushed away all the things that would have helped me, my behaviour became confusing and upsetting for the people around me. As I felt their reaction, I would distance myself further, which only resulted in more isolation and drinking. I had effectively decided to administer my own medicine in the form of a lot of booze, which wasn't helping me; it was just making me sicker. There might be a day or moments when I would pull it together 'to keep the wheels moving' if I had something I needed to do for work, but mostly I was stuck in a downward spiral. In fact, at that time, even if I did understand what was happening, I didn't know how to stop it.

In other words, the whole thing was slow and painful – my bathtub was gradually filling with water. Looking back now, there was a scary inevitability about it, as BANG! that one extra drop of water landed in my bathtub and it was all too much; I was overwhelmed with darkness all around me.

The most basic things in life felt utterly impossible. I couldn't get out of bed; I was terrified to speak to anyone; I couldn't answer my phone. I went from being a high-performing human being to a door mat. I had landed in an extremely dark and unmanageable mental place, and the process from start to finish probably took six months.

There is part of me that has wondered whether I have pressed the 'fuck-it' button – as in, decided to ignore what is healthy for me and get into damaging behaviours – in those situations because I have led a very disciplined life with gymnastics, so when a reason comes for me to be free with my behaviour, I let loose. But, you know what? That's an excuse. I could throw myself into a million different things that are healthy that I am not able to do when I can't train full time. I could hang out with friends, read books, listen to podcasts, go for walks and watch films for 12 hours a day! The reason I went into isolation and alcohol is because I hadn't learned how to sit with the physical and mental pain that I was in. I didn't have the tools to deal with it and went for the easy option – escape. This is why I describe this process as being one of compounding decisions. That first decision I make, which doesn't feel like a disaster at the time, starts off a chain of events that ultimately leads to very poor mental health.

If this slide happens to you and you've never experienced it before, then you'll probably have no idea what's going on.

You won't spot the pattern or even the direction of travel, and it is as confusing for you as it is for others. But what if it's not your first time and you have an inkling of what's happening? Can you stop it, and if you don't, why not?

These are great questions for me because I have definitely been in situations that I knew were only heading one way but I couldn't pull myself out of it. But I do believe that it is possible to get yourself off that slide. By first recognising what's going and then using certain tools or methods that I'll talk you through in this book, you can get yourself back to a healthier place. So then why on earth would you choose not to do this?

Unfortunately I have done this far too many times. When you're on a downward spiral and you're at least partially aware of it, your self-esteem can take a massive hit. I know that I am making poor decisions in those moments and begin to feel really shit about myself. I recognise that I am letting myself fall into that hole again. It almost feels worse knowing some of this stuff rather than being completely oblivious to it. I beat myself up for making rubbish decisions, which just leads to more rubbish decisions. I know that none of it is rational, and that's the problem with mental health issues – you can't seem to differentiate between what is rational and irritational. The thoughts all feel the same.

When I am beating myself up like this, I develop this strange thought pattern that says, 'Well, I might as well properly fuck this up now!' I guess it's because it's what I think I deserve. My mind tells me that because I have got myself into a mess, *again*, that I deserve nothing short of a massive crash. One bad thought creates the next bad thought, and before you know it, you're in a really dark place. You want better for yourself and everyone around you, but, fundamentally, you feel out of control and it's incredibly scary.

Writing this chapter has been a great reminder of how difficult it is for the loved ones of someone who is struggling with their mental health. Yes, it is deeply confusing and difficult for those suffering, but for the people who just want to help, it can feel equally impossible to manage. First and foremost, this is because the person they love begins to behave in ways that can upset, annoy or confuse them.

As an example, I love nothing more than laughing and spending time with my family. We have always been a really social family and I have loved being in the middle of it, whether it's at the golf club with my dad or at the pub with my whole family. We bounce off each other and share such positive energy. But then, as I slide into a dark place with my mental health, I totally change. I don't want to spend time with them. I don't want to know what's going on in their lives. I withdraw from them almost entirely. For my family, this is deeply upsetting because it's not who we are. We pride ourselves on supporting each other with whatever

we are doing, and yet then I present to them as being completely self-absorbed and uninterested in them. When I'm
completely lost in my own head, I just appear to be really
selfish – but I don't mean it like that. I can't get out of my
own destructive thoughts at that moment in time. I barely
have enough energy to cope with myself, let alone socialise
with other people, even people I love.

That's why the fall is incredibly difficult for people around
you, and it also comes from a compounding effect. Over
time, as you push them away, their confusion, frustration
and anger builds, until your relationship with them is in a
bad place. Initially, they can tell you're not your normal self
and want to know why. For me, the challenge is that when I
am asked that, I don't really have a coherent answer because
I am trying to work it out myself. Someone who simply
wants to help you can feel useless in that moment. As I withdraw more, they try harder; my behaviour becomes more
confusing, they try even harder; I withdraw even more and,
eventually, they get fed up with me – and I can understand
why! I could be sitting with my family for two hours and not
ask them a single question about what's going on in their
lives, while I give them nothing meaningful to understand
how I am. As I become aware of the impact I am having on
them, it's one more thing to beat myself up over, another
reason to think I am a shit person who deserves to be in a

mess, and the compounding continues. It is such a destructive pattern or cycle to be stuck in.

It's also really important to acknowledge how destructive the alcohol element is within all this. If I have been feeling and behaving the way I have described, but then go on big booze binges where I look like I'm having a good time, what are my family meant to think? I just look like a self-centred, spoilt brat. Alcohol can have me smiling, laughing and messing around when I am actually in a really dark place mentally – it creates a completely contradictory message. My parents have seen me the day after a big night out when I am extremely hungover and struggling mentally, but to them I just look like someone who has overindulged and is now feeling sorry for themselves. If frustration is at an all-time high then it's so hard for them to remain patient with me. If I ask for help at that moment in time you can see how they would second guess whether it was me or just the hangover speaking. Sadly, it's a pattern that can ruin relationships.

I hope my experiences have served as a good example of how deteriorating mental health comes from a compounding effect of thoughts, decisions and actions. It's so important to understand that it is multi-layered and, as a result, requires some unravelling. This book is very much about presenting solutions to you to help you with your mental health;

however, an important starting point is to understand what you are dealing with. These solutions lie in reversing or, even better, preventing that slide from beginning in the first place.

In the next chapter, I want to talk you through the close connection between addiction and mental health issues for the same reason. Understanding this link doesn't necessarily present you with an immediate solution, but it gives you an all-important insight into the traps that we fall into and why. This has been absolutely key for me and I feel it's crucial to unpack it. If I had understood what I am going to tell you in the next chapter a few years ago, it would have saved me a lot of pain along the way.

HAVING TO FACE REALITY

I've been an addict all my life. My pa sometimes reminds me about when I was a kid and he would read me a bedtime story. A child wanting a bedtime story is perfectly normal, but the thing that was unusual was that I used to make him read exactly the same book every single night for months on end. I would fall in love with one particular story and become fixated on it. I couldn't get enough of it, until I could no longer keep my eyes open.

It was this level of obsession that meant I got immediately hooked on gymnastics at four years old. It was an instant addiction to learning and perfecting new skills, as well as performing and competing. The same applied to creating content on YouTube. I have been addicted to creating videos that go viral and entertain millions of people. This tendency to addiction has been one of my greatest strengths as well as one of my greatest weaknesses in life. At its best, it has driven me to making Olympic history in gymnastics; at its worst, it has driven me to lose tens of thousands of pounds in a week and having to be forcibly banned from all the casinos in the UK.

So it's fair to say that I have been on a journey with addiction – one on which I have learned a great deal. I want to share my experiences with you because I know how important finally understanding them has been to my mental health. This chapter is not about me preaching to you about how to solve addiction issues, not at all; it is simply me helping you to connect the dots between addictive behaviour and poor mental health. Understanding this connection has the power to help transform someone's life, and that might be the case for you.

For me, addiction is when I lose all control over the thing I am doing and it has total power over me. The pull of it is so intense that it feels inevitable. I might pretend to people around me and to myself that it is a choice, but it isn't. During my worst gambling days, I would tell people that I *wanted* to go to the casino or gamble online, but that was total bollocks. The urge drawing me towards it was overwhelming, suffocating and relentless. I knew I shouldn't be doing it; I knew it was bad for me; I knew it would take me to even worse places. And yet, I still did it. Gambling at that time was controlling me, not the other way around.

It wasn't just the lure to start doing it; it was also what

happened once I started. I didn't know where it would end up or stop. It was like being stuck in a vortex that would decide when it was ready to chuck me out. Betting companies and casinos make enormous profits because the vast majority of gamblers lose over a long period of time, and I was no different – yet I was stuck in a loop I had no idea how to get out of. In the cold light of day, that's terrifying. I couldn't decide that enough was enough for that night, day, week or month. That is a feeling of being completely powerless. That is addiction for me.

I have often been asked and wondered myself whether poor mental health leads to addiction difficulties or vice versa. I have come to believe that it doesn't really matter. What I do know is that they are very closely related. They work hand-in-hand to take you down a very dark hole. The key point for me now is to understand why this is the case, rather than trying to unpick which leads the other. Difficulties with addiction, just like other mental health issues, creep up on you. They are also bloody sneaky buggers! They very slowly walk you towards a place that, when you get there, you can't believe you have arrived in.

I'm going to talk you through how this can happen, step by step, and I want you to pause throughout it to self-reflect. Do you recognise this process? Have you felt the same feelings and developed some of these same coping mechanisms that I did? There will be differences in our experiences, of course – we are all in different situations and have different personalities – but look for the similarities in emotions. Developing this understanding of yourself is going to be key in helping you get as much as possible from this book.

The best analogy I can give is this – imagine if after the first time you picked up a beer you lost your job, your partner left you, you got arrested, you crashed your car, you were humiliated, you began getting health issues and experiencing acute depression and low self-esteem. You would *never* drink alcohol again! But it doesn't do that to you, unfortunately. It quietly and gently convinces you that it is a solution to some of your problems. It appears to fix your stress, bring you happiness and fun, even improve your friendships – it's *your* friend. Why wouldn't you go along for the ride with it? The upside looks way better than the downside. So, you start this friendship – in this case with alcohol – and like any 'good' friendship, it grows. You become closer. Alcohol makes you happier so why wouldn't you hook up more?! It all makes perfect sense. But then . . . it doesn't. Very slowly, something changes. Suddenly, alcohol doesn't make you happier, it makes you sad. It used to calm your nerves but now you get crippling anxiety. You loved drinking with your friends and being social, and now you want to be on your own drinking in the kitchen. What. The. Hell. Happened?

But now here comes the real kicker to this whole thing.

This has been a close relationship that has developed over a long time. For most of that time, it's been great. It's only now that it seems to be a problem. So, at this moment in time, your mind tells you that the problem can't be the alcohol. It is your most loyal and trusted friend, after all! It has to be something else. It's your job, your lack of job, your relationship, your lack of relationship, your stress, your lack of stress, your purpose, your lack of purpose – just anything, goddamn it! So you don't move away from your friend; in fact, quite the opposite, you move closer towards it – 'it will save me, as it always has!' What you don't realise right now is that you have just handed over all control to your friend, alcohol.

While you slide into a dark place in life due to your reliance on alcohol, your love of it has created a level of denial that means you stay stuck in this hole. It's like drowning underwater and telling yourself that water would never do this to you, so you swim even deeper. It's madness but it happens. You might read all of this and think that I have got the whole thing sussed out – well, I haven't. I know what danger there is in these sorts of patterns, but I still need to watch myself on a daily basis.

So, how does this all link to how we manage our mental health?

I'm sure by now you can see how similar the processes are of declining mental health and increasing addiction issues.

They are both slow and subtle. While you think you are in control of what you are doing, they are very subtly taking that control away from you. The steps you take to get into those dark places are part of that compounding effect that I talked about in the last chapter. However, hands down the biggest reason for me that addiction and deteriorating mental health are so intrinsically linked is because they both involve me not being prepared to face and deal with the reality of my feelings at that time. This has been an enormous learning for me and one that I am continually working on.

If I experience something difficult, for example my neck injury, I immediately face challenges to my mental stability because I feel physical and mental pain. That's completely understandable and would be pretty much the same for everyone. Feeling anxious, panicked or unsure of yourself is a perfectly standard human reaction to something that really upsets your world. Can you look back on moments in your life when you have felt this sort of mental instability after something has happened to you? Often we feel it the most intensely when it is completely unexpected. If, in this sort of moment, I haven't been looking after myself with good daily habits up to that point then I can be particularly vulnerable to instability. But now is the crucial bit.

It's all about how I handle this situation, and the word FEAR sums it all up. Do I . . . ?

FEAR – Fuck everything and run!

FEAR – Face everything and rise!

Take a moment now to think through how you have reacted in the sorts of challenging situations that you have just reflected on. Did you run or did you face everything? I have had to ask myself these difficult questions. This has been an incredibly difficult learning for me because, for a long time, I didn't realise how dominated by fear I actually was. 'I'm an Olympian, business owner, YouTuber etc', 'I'm not scared of anything' is what I would tell myself. But that was a lie. I was scared – really scared. I have learned that I have been terrified of my feelings for much of my life. Fear has gripped me whenever I haven't liked how I was feeling and I have reacted to that by running away from it. Option one was my only way of doing things for long time because I didn't even know there was an alternative.

When I have started on that slide, when I haven't been looking after myself and I've allowed unhealthy habits to creep into my life then my mental health slowly deteriorates. Not only do I not want to feel like that, I don't want to face why I am feeling like that. That's too hard. Instead, I just want to run away from it all – I want ESCAPE. Alcohol and gambling have proved to be brilliant escape plans because they distract me, they numb me, they take me away from . . . guess who? ME! And, as I have already described, those things seem like they are my best friends in that moment, but, inevitably, they start to turn against me and make things

31

worse. As this happens, I want more escape and I keep going back to my 'friends', thinking that they will keep saving me from my feelings. The vicious cycle has begun and I am completely powerless once again.

The above paints a picture of what leads to addiction issues for me, but it can work the other way round as well. I might be in a good or OK place with my mental health, but then addiction issues raise their heads and send me on that downwards slide. Alcohol and gambling are not healthy for me – they isolate me, they take me away from looking after my physical health, they mess with my sleeping patterns, and I feel shame and regret for my behaviour when I am doing them. All of which puts me back in the same spot, wanting to run away from how I feel. Before I know it, I'm stuck in the same bloody process!

I hope you can now see how intertwined mental health and addiction issues are. They can feed each other. Sometimes one leads and the other follows, and sometimes the other way around, but they are always close by. Making the connection between that behaviour pattern and the end result has been huge for me.

So, what are the answers to all this? Well, it comes down to option two above: **FEAR – Face everything and rise!**

I have had to learn – or, more accurately, I am still learning – to 'sit with pain'. What I mean by 'pain' is any feeling that I basically don't like! This can be severe anxiety or something simple like boredom. And by 'sitting with it', I mean not doing anything significant to distract me from that feeling so I recognise and feel all of it. I have found this *so* hard! Every part of me wants to escape feelings that I don't like. Is this something you can relate to?

Let's look at what I mean by starting with something relatively simple: boredom. There's nothing wrong with being bored, right? Of course not! Boredom is perfectly normal. However, feeling bored or even not wanting to feel bored has led to so many problems for me.

Before I get into that, though, I want to explain what I mean by 'boredom'. It can come from not having anything to do or needing to do something that I don't enjoy, but it can also come from tranquillity. Yes, believe it or not, I can get uncomfortable when everything feels too calm! And the reason for that is actually really key to understanding what's going on in my head. I can feel uncomfortable with tranquillity because it often leaves me with myself and my own thoughts. In other words, if I am sitting in my flat with no problems on the horizon but also nothing to distract me, then it's just me and my thoughts and I find that really hard. In fact, I have hated it and have just wanted to get away from it.

Why? I'm not sure but it's a pattern that I have always had. It feels like my immediate response to silence is an overwhelming need for stimulation of some sort in order to get away from that silence. I'm sure that a lot or all of you can relate to that in some way. It's probably linked to our constant desire to check our phones every millisecond. But consider this in other situations:

Have there been times within a relationship that it has felt too calm for you?

Do you find it excruciating when there is a pause for silence when chatting to friends?

I have definitely felt those things. The difficulty, though, is that this can lead to the start of an unhealthy pattern. Essentially, I am triggering a response within me to distract myself or escape from reality. I can't handle just sitting with my thoughts in peace so I run away. If I distract myself with something like alcohol or gambling then I start all the processes that are going to cause me to slide down to a dark place. And all because I didn't want to sit with my feelings. Crazy, really.

What I have described also exists on the other end of the scale, when I am really struggling with crippling anxiety. It can be so horrible with every part of my being wanting to get away from it, but I've learned that my answer can't be to try to escape from the reality of it. I need to sit with that pain and do healthy things that will help cure it rather than ignore it. It's like having an injury and simply reaching for a temporary painkiller rather than actually trying to do things to heal the injury. When you don't heal it, it keeps returning *and* gets worse and worse. That's why the option of FEAR – face everything and rise, has to always be the one I choose, however difficult and painful that is, because on the other side of it is healing.

Are there things in your life that you are running from because you are scared of dealing with them and they continue to haunt you? Or have you faced something, as difficult as it was, and come out the other side feeling healed from it? These could be difficult conversations, relationships, decisions or past experiences. Take some time now to consider this.

If this is brand new to you then remember that it can take time to learn how to do it and you don't perfect it overnight. It might even feel painful to begin with, but don't panic; sometimes growth can feel like that, but the end result will be huge personal progress. I am very much a 'work in progress' and here are the key tools that help me. I would love you to try these out, rather than searching for a distraction, when you are uncomfortable with your feelings:

Meditation

This is the literal version of you sitting in silence with your thoughts. I have found meditation really hard at times, as my mind races with what feels like a million thoughts a minute. But every time I commit to it, I feel the benefit of learning to sit with myself, even if it is just for five or ten minutes. One crucial element to this, which I am reminded about a lot, is that meditation isn't a test. It's not something where you have to 'do it right'; it is simply a practice. So, by trying it regularly, you are already winning. You don't need to be 'good' at it. The more you practise, the easier it will become. Don't judge yourself on how you think it went, but rather by how consistently you are doing it.

Talk to someone

You don't have to sit alone with your feelings, especially when they are difficult ones. By sharing them with someone else through talking or messaging then you are not running away from them; in fact, you are addressing them head on. We can have this illusion in our heads that we need to fix everything ourselves and we shouldn't burden anyone else with our problems. That is not at all true, and being open about your feelings to someone else can lift a huge weight off your shoulders.

Get some exercise

Some of my best thinking time comes when I exercise, and I will be talking more about this later. When we exercise we often clear space in our head because some of our attention is needed to keep our body moving. This takes us to a much calmer headspace, allowing us to think things through and let feelings sit with us. Going for a run when you feel angry is not a bad idea at all. It doesn't mean you forget you are angry, but while you are outdoors and moving, you have some time to let that emotion sit and the space to calm down.

Get outside into nature

When I'm stuck inside the walls of my apartment my thoughts can feel overwhelming, but when I get outside into nature, they can be brought so much more into perspective. Those nagging worries often suddenly feel so much less important when I see the size and beauty of nature. Importantly, this doesn't mean that I am escaping from my thoughts, but rather that I have more power to find a clearer perspective around them. Also, feeling fresh air in my lungs and breathing properly helps me to calm my nervous system.

Listen to music or a podcast

Again, this isn't about distracting yourself; it's about creating a headspace environment that allows you to sit more comfortably with your feelings. Music can calm me, move me and allow me to breathe some perspective into whatever it is that is rattling around in my head. Because I know now that I struggle with tranquillity and want to fill that space. I can see that a little bit of music or background talking allows me to think much more calmly and fill the silence in a way that is healthy.

Write it down

I would always try to speak to someone first to share how I was feeling, but if that's not possible, for whatever reason, then writing down how you feel can be so helpful. I find that by having to think through what words to write I start to make sense of my feelings. It does feel like an unburdening. Some people will journal a lot, which is great, but that has never really been me. Scribbling down some thoughts on a scrap of paper works just as well for me in those moments when I need it.

Learning to sit with your feelings and emotions is tough, but it's made infinitely easier by asking for help from others. Yet asking for help can seem incredibly difficult when you feel vulnerable with your mental health. What would appear to be a simple action feels like nothing of the sort in those moments. In this next chapter, I will give you some practical tools to make this easier for you, particularly when your mental health is not at its best.

I'M NOT ALRIGHT, MATE

Asking for help should be an easy thing to do, right? Surely it's a human instinct when we're in trouble? I just picture in my mind a caveman running away from a terrifying animal, screaming for help. It's a primal reaction, so why do we sometimes find it so hard to do this when we are struggling with our mental health? What are the blocks that stop us reaching out and instead leave us in that dark and lonely place?

It's a really important question, as the truth is that it's so hard to improve your mental health and get out of that hole unless you are able to ask for help. So let's start with the 'why' we find it hard to reach out for help, as understanding this is a crucial first step towards finding solutions. Then I'm going to give you some really simple ways to overcome this, if it is something you struggle with.

Reason 1: We have no idea what's going on

The first reason we can find asking for help so difficult relates back to the things we have just been discussing – mental health challenges bloody creep up on you! The decline we experience is so slow and subtle that we can't work out how we've ended up in the place that we are. This confusion is a massive reason why people find it difficult to ask for help, and even more so if these sorts of challenges are relatively new to them. You don't actually know what you should be asking for help *for* because it's hard to understand what's happening to you. It's why the whole thing can be so isolating for someone, because you are trying to work out things in real time when you feel like a completely different person.

I have often felt like I didn't know how to explain the way I was feeling, so I just wouldn't bother starting. But there are more layers to this. The thoughts going through my head in dark times make ABSOLUTELY NO SENSE! For example, I'm a young man with a great family, amazing friends, money, success . . . and yet I can feel like my world is imploding and I am completely useless. None of it adds up, especially not to me. I have that conversation with myself, saying, 'What have I got to feel sad or depressed about?! Pull yourself together!' I beat myself up about how crazy it all seems. And if I can't make sense of it then how do I explain it to someone else and ask for their help? It can feel impossible.

Reason 2: We expect to be able to fix everything by ourselves

This is going to sound specific to myself, or at least elite sportspeople, but I feel that it relates to everyone to some degree. My entire life in gymnastics has been about mastering something until it's as close to perfect as it can be. Gymnasts are used to failure – we will practise a skill 100 times and get it wrong 99 times just for that single success. My life has been built around accepting what's going wrong and quickly finding a solution to get on the road to success. I have backed that up with constantly talking positively to myself; in the Olympic final, I even screamed 'I can do this!' just before I started my routine. I have always believed that the mindset needed to conquer things is part of my DNA. I've always viewed it as a key part of who I am as a person. I don't get downhearted when I get something wrong, I just rapidly click into finding a solution and move forwards again.

Now, I understand that this part of me is at an extreme level compared to people not in elite performance, but that doesn't mean no one else feels it too. On a basic level, we see problem-solving as part of being an independent adult – we want to sort stuff out! We think we should know what to do and be able to stand on our own two feet. Different people take different amounts of time to find solutions in their lives, but it is part of being a human being. We don't keep putting our hand in the fire because we learn that it will burn us.

Well, mental health issues throw an absolute spanner in the works for all this!

My life has been about 'fixing' things. Fixing imperfections in a gymnastics routine, figuring out how to make money on YouTube, even fairly recently learning how to ice skate for *Dancing on Ice*! So much of what I have done has been built around getting over or through obstacles, but then – BANG! I couldn't find a solution for how I was feeling in my head. Nothing made sense, I didn't know how I had got where I had and, most importantly, I didn't know how to get out of there. Suddenly, I had no answers. A lifelong fixer was completely lost. A huge part of my identity had been built around me succeeding and now I couldn't.

Has this ever been you? Have you ever run into a problem you had no idea how to solve, or even figure out the source of, and it's knocked you for six?

No one likes feeling useless and helpless, and that is exactly what poor mental health can do to you. I have wanted to 'fix' it myself because admitting that I can't felt like letting go of part of who I was as a person. For a long period of time, I would rather have drowned inside my own head's thoughts than ask someone for help, as back to front as that sounds.

Reason 3: We don't know who to ask for help

The third reason we struggle to ask for help is that we don't know *who* to speak to. You have a problem that you can't really explain and think you'll sound stupid talking about it, and then you have to find a person who you think might understand – that can be really hard!

I believe that this can particularly apply to men. We are just not as good at talking about our feelings as women are, and especially not with other men. This is in no way to take away from the challenges that many women have in speaking about their mental health, everyone is different, but I do believe that, on the whole, us men find this really tricky. As an example, I found this hard not just because I didn't talk to my mates about this sort of thing, but also because I was aware of how they saw me. They saw me as a confident Olympian, an over-achiever, an elite athlete who had all the answers to everything. They didn't see me as someone who struggled and, crucially, I didn't *want* them to see me as someone who struggled. It was no one's fault and not a reflection on my family or friends, but it meant that I didn't always want to tell them how I was truly feeling. I think a lot of us struggle with this when we first experience problems with our mental health – if we're not already in the habit of being open (and sometimes even if we are) then there isn't always an obvious outlet for us that feels safe.

Reason 4: We feel embarrassed

The final reason why people struggle to reach out is shame. Yeah, that's right, shame or embarrassment or guilt – or all of them muddled together. It can come from a sense that we should have sorted this out by now on our own and we don't want to burden anyone else with our issues. If we are still trying to understand our mental health challenges then we can sometimes tell ourselves that we are failing by not sorting them out without help from others. The conversation in society around mental health has moved forward massively in the last ten years. I wouldn't be writing this book if it hadn't, and I am really grateful for that on a number of levels. But that doesn't mean to say that it feels completely judgement free. There is nothing necessarily sinister about this, though, it's just a lack of education on the subject. I'm a young lad in Leeds and it's still not the sort of thing that people of my age are talking about in pubs and clubs.

The fact is that mental illness is hidden inside your head; it's not a broken bone that people can see, you don't look unwell and like you need to be in hospital. And with anything that is invisible, there will be some people who understand it and others who don't, especially among young people. That is not a slate against people who don't get it, because I can see that it is difficult to do so if you've not experienced it. In fact, I was that person before I started to have my own struggles. I believed that if you told yourself positive things enough times, you would always stay positive! And then depression and anxiety came along and absolutely cornered me. It has also been so hard for my family to come to terms with it all. They haven't had the same issues so they've understandably needed time to learn about what was going on with me.

Like I've said, we live in a society in which there is far greater understanding of mental health issues but not a *uniform* understanding. It is in these gaps of misunderstanding where shame can exist for a sufferer. The shame comes from being embarrassed about feeling the way they do, because the message they are getting is that their feelings are not real and they need to 'pull themselves together'. That's a horrible place to be in. The peak example of this is if you have grown up in a house where people have said to you that mental health issues are a load of nonsense and made up by 'weak' people. If you are surrounded by that and then begin suffering with it, why would you even try to reach out for help? Keeping it locked in your head would feel like a far better option.

So, reaching out for help can be much harder for some than others, and maybe still much harder than it should be in an ideal world. Do you relate to that? Have there been moments in your life when you have desperately needed help but found that you couldn't get yourself to reach out for it? Do you know which of the reasons above were the biggest barrier for you? Let's now focus on how we can turn this around.

You don't need to have all the answers yourself

It's so important to remember that you don't have to be able to explain clearly what is going on when you reach out for help. In the hot mess of the feelings in our heads, we can tell ourselves that we need to be able to make sense of it all before we can talk to someone else – that is NOT true! In actual fact, that is part of the problem. In not wanting to sound 'weird', I ended up not saying anything at all for ages. You do not need to make sense when you reach out for help!

I'll give you my example of this. I have always had a really open relationship with my manager, Luke, and can tell him pretty much anything. In 2018, I was driving to Lilleshall in Shropshire to meet up with the Great Britain squad for a training camp. I had been struggling with injuries but, more importantly, just with coping with life. I felt hopeless and lost. I didn't know who I was anymore and felt terrified about having to go into a training camp, which previously I had adored. I had always loved being around the squad, but everything felt different now.

I was desperate. I didn't know how to express what I was feeling, but still I called Luke. Through tears and a lot of snot, I just blurted stuff out. None of it came out in any order or made any sense – it was just a release of desperation. He later said that he'd never heard me speak that way. He called the Team GB doctor immediately after we hung up to plan how they could put support in place for me. I look back on that and realise that it was a great learning point for me: I reached out for help but not in any well-worded or fancy way. I just blurted it out – snot and all – and it was heard. That's all we need.

You can start by writing stuff down to help you make sense of it

I'm no great writer – which might be what you're thinking as you read this book, ha-ha! I don't really write much down in journals or diaries; I don't have a special notebook that I carry around to record my thoughts or track how I feel. Which is a bit of a shame, as I actually think it would be really beneficial for me – but it's just not me. I'm a visual person, which is why I have always loved talking to camera on YouTube rather than writing. But having said all this, I do understand the powerful impact of writing in sorting out the jumble in your head. Give it a go anyway, but particularly if you feel you are still working up to talking to another human about what's going on for you.

Asking for help can be as simple as a five-word text

Even though I haven't written anything regularly or in any kind of structured way, I have written crucial messages to people when I have needed them. I'll give you some examples of things I have written to my friends and family when I've been in a dark place.

'I'm not alright, mate.'

'I don't want to be alone.'

'I don't feel in a great place.'

'Can you come around to mine?'

'I'm not good.'

Not much, hey? They are really short and don't explain anything other than I need support. This is what a reach out for help can look like. It doesn't need to be an essay; it can be as simple as this. Sending a short message can feel much easier than having to actually speak to someone, but the person receiving it will understand that you need help. Five or six words in a message can be powerful enough.

Talking about it makes it normal

It's not like this is going to be top of your to-do list if you find yourself in a dark place, but the truth is that educating people who don't understand mental health is particularly important. Try to talk about your mental health regularly to friends and members of your family who you feel comfortable with. By the way, it doesn't always have to be negative!

Tell them when you're feeling great and how that compares to when you are feeling in a dark place. Give them a barometer to work off. That could be something as simple as a score out of ten. Help them to see why, on one day, you are an eight out of ten, and on another, you are a two out of ten. With the right info they'll learn to see the signs when you're doing well and those when you're struggling.

The more you talk about and describe your mental health, the more you are helping others to understand and be able to help you when you need it. You are also creating a space where it feels safe to talk about it openly, and that's invaluable in the long term, for other people and the wider conversation too. The shame and awkwardness around it gets lifted and we all start talking about it in the same way we would if someone was recovering from a physical injury. Greater understanding means greater ease for the conversation. And it's within your power to have a positive impact there.

Find your safe space

The final point I want to make about breaking down the barriers that stop us from talking about how we feel and asking for help links heavily to what I have said above. It's crucial to have or find a safe space in which you feel comfortable to reach out for help when you need it. I am lucky that I have people in my life who have suffered with mental health issues before I did, so they were obvious people for me to reach out to, but I have also experienced reaching out to people with less knowledge of these issues and it has gone really badly. I know how hard this can be, so it is *so* important that you search out for people or communities that represent safety for you.

The reality is that there will be people around you all the time who are suffering with mental health issues. You might not know it but they are there. Since I have started speaking publicly about my own difficulties, so many people I know have approached me about their own challenges. I knew nothing of their issues, but by speaking out, I guess I helped create a safe space for them to talk to me.

One of the most brilliant people I know in gymnastics is my old Great Britain coach, Barry Collie. 'Baz' and I energised each other in the gym, and anything seemed possible with him. He challenged me and I challenged him, but we loved it – it was like there was a brightly burning spark between us that brought out brilliance in the gym. I fucking loved it. I used to look forward to my sessions with Baz so much! I trained with him for around ten years and went on multiple trips away with him to competitions. We were and are super close, and yet it has only been in the last year or so that he has opened up to me about his issues with addiction and mental health.

It's like it forms a chain: someone created a safe space for me and then in turn I created one for Baz – I love that. So, you have to get pro-active and look for your own safe spaces. If there is someone in your life you are already close to who you can talk to – like I did with my manager Luke – that's great, but if you can't think of anyone don't give up! You can also look online. There are so many people talking about mental health in online communities now. They are there and you are not alone.

Ultimately, poor mental health isolates you. It makes you want to curl up in a little ball and talk to no one. It can be an incredibly self-absorbing experience. You can't see beyond yourself because your feelings are suffocating you. But when you find your person or people to reach out to, you can break this a little. All you have to say is 'I'm not alright, mate' and that's enough. A bridge has been formed. It can also work the other way around when you're feeling shit. If, in that moment, you can find the strength to ask someone how they are, then you move away from thinking about how bad you feel by focusing on someone else's feelings. Another bridge has been formed and you can then help each other. The thing is that humans need humans, humans love humans – we just need to create that connection with each other.

Before we head into the next chapter, I want to make an important point. Sometimes it can feel like mental health issues are happening *to* us, and that is true to some extent, but I hope you have started to see how often the idea of personal responsibility comes up in everything that I have said so far. There are actions very much within our control that can help us enormously with our mental health. We have to recognise what *we* can do, and that is very much where we are going in this next chapter.

WHY WE KEEP FUCKING UP

I have always seen myself as an honest person. My ma and pa encouraged my sister, Joanna, and I to be open and truthful about our feelings and share what we are doing – the good and the bad. In fact, sometimes friends would be shocked about how honest we are with our parents! However, my mental health challenges have forced me to reassess my whole relationship with honesty. This isn't about lying to people; it's about whether I am always being honest with myself. I have learned that to stay healthy I need to face up to what I do to help myself and, more importantly, what I'm not doing to help myself.

A mental health decline can be full of patterns of behaviour that are harming you. Recognising and then stopping these destructive patterns is so important, but it does usually require us to face uncomfortable truths. If we live in denial about what we're doing then we have little or zero chance of stopping them.

I'm going to talk more about self-destructive patterns and what they are, but, before I get further into it, does this sound familiar at all? If I asked you to come up with two or three things you tend to do when you are feeling shit that, if you're being honest, don't help or have particularly great outcomes, what would you say?

To be fair, I didn't even know such things as self-destructive patterns existed until it was broken down for me. Let's start with this – every feeling can trigger a thought and every thought can trigger an action. For example, I feel hungry (feeling), I should get some food (thought), I find food (action). Feelings are non-negotiable – we feel what we feel – but thoughts sit in between them and the eventual action. When you consider this you can see that actions are dominated by thoughts. I might tell myself that I am suddenly doing something without really thinking about it, but a thought will have come before it. Let me give you three examples from my life.

1. I feel unstable and out of control

As a result, I think that I need to find stability in my life. Eventually, I end up getting into a relationship that I hope is going to give me stability. Have I got myself into a relationship for the right reasons? No. It was an action that was created because of an initial feeling of instability and then a conscious or subconscious thought that stability lay in a relationship with this person. As that relationship inevitably breaks down, I can tell myself that 'it wasn't meant to be' or I can delve deeper and uncover the true motivation behind what led me to that point.

2. I feel like I have let down people who are close to me

I can give you a specific example of this, actually – my sister was working in corporate hospitality at Headingley cricket ground in 2019 when England were playing Australia in the Ashes. Joanna managed to get free tickets with full hospitality for me, my two mates and my dad. It was such a treat for us all and we were supposed to arrive at 10am. I turned up about an hour and a half late and incredibly hungover, having had about three hours' sleep. As soon as I walked in, I saw my sister and dad's reaction and felt like I'd let them down. As a result, I started to think about how useless I was instead of being the person that I should be to them. That led to me having a 'pity party' as I self-loathed. So, stuck on the thought that I was no good to anyone, I just start drinking again. Reasonable reaction? No. This makes things a million times worse.

3. I feel disliked

Because one of my old friends doesn't greet me as enthusiastically as I think he should when I see him. I think that he must not like me anymore for some reason, and I hate that. As a result, I decide to blank him going forward because I don't want him to do that to me again. I convince myself that it is him who's the dickhead now and I want to keep him away from me. Does this make rational sense? No. I have no idea what's going on in his life and have just hooked onto an immediate feeling based on how I *expected* he should react to me. By pushing him away, I am then acting like the dickhead rather than just talking to him and seeing how he is.

These are situations that directly affect my mental health, and they all start with a feeling and then a thought and then a self-destructive action. If it keeps happening, then it is a self-destructive pattern. I have had to learn this from the bottom up. For a very long time, I would just blame everyone and everything else rather than facing my uncomfortable truths. I just didn't know that I was lying to myself and I was in denial about why I behaved in certain ways.

OK, now it's your turn to play detective. I challenge you to think about an unhealthy situation that you get yourself into or an unreasonable reaction.

Can you trace it back to an initial feeling that gave you the thought that triggered the action? There will be something there.

How often does this happen to you and how does it affect your mental health?

You might be surprised by the results. This is where mental health issues are not happening *to* us, but are being *created* by us. This has been a hard realisation for me to accept.

There are a ton of other examples that I could give you, but I really want us to focus on how we learn to stop these sorts of patterns taking hold in our lives. Before I start talking you through what I have learned, I need you to remember that this is literally a 're-training' of your brain. You might have been unknowingly stuck in these patterns for years or even decades. You are not going to fix this in five minutes or even a week. It's going to take regular practice and you're going to fuck it up a few times. And when you do, you'll need to take a deep breath, chalk it up to experience and try again. The important thing is that you stay aware of it and you keep trying to stop it before it takes you down a really bad path.

I hope that you have understood the point I made about our feelings leading to thoughts and our thoughts leading to actions. I would suggest reading back over it if you just want to solidify the point in your mind. By the way, I make this all sound simple, but, honestly, it took me a long time to get my head around it! Ultimately, if we are to recognise and stop self-destructive patterns then we have to be on top of this chain from feeling to action.

Let's take a moment to acknowledge how powerful our

feelings are. One feeling alone can spark such a negative reaction that it ends in an action that can really harm us. It's mad when you think about it like that.

As a gymnast, I thrived off emotion and atmosphere. It inspired me and gave me energy. I wasn't some sort of robot just going through a mechanical process to win a medal, I was full of feelings. The euphoric high of an Olympics Games was very real for me. I felt every ounce of adrenaline pumping through my body as I performed in front of the world – it was magical. But all this has another side to it: while I can be inspired by positive feelings, I can also be crippled by negative feelings. I can be suffocated by anxiety while I worry about what someone thinks of me or whether I have done the right thing in a certain situation.

The easiest example I can give you to illustrate this was when I spoke out publicly in 2020 about the culture of abuse that existed in British gymnastics at the time. It was in the aftermath of the *Athlete A* documentary on Netflix, which showed everyone the unthinkable abuse that young gymnasts had suffered in the US. I have been blessed to have had some incredible coaches, but I felt it was the right time to highlight the huge issues within the sport in our country. However, the cost to my mental health was massive. As much as many people supported me within gymnastics, there were many who didn't want me to speak out about the inconvenient truth that existed then in our sport. The split of opinion was made immediately obvious by reading comments online and via friends within the gymnastics community. I felt it all. I couldn't help getting anxious about whether I was losing friends and if people were talking about me behind my back. That worry grew into full-blown anxiety and depression. Despite doing something I felt was vital for the sport I loved so much, I ended up being in a dark place for weeks after it. If what I am describing here resonates with you, then don't underestimate how powerfully your feelings can drive you in both positive and negative ways.

My next talking point actually blows my mind. I appreciate this might be a little tricky to understand immediately, but bear with me. Sometimes the thoughts generated from our feelings are not actually real. But thoughts are thoughts, right? How can they not be real? Well, a huge discovery for me has been that this isn't true, but if I allow them to grow in my mind then they will become my reality.

Let me show you using one of my examples above: 'I feel like I have let down people who are close to me.' As a result, I think that I'm useless and not the person that I should be to them. I have absolutely done this in the past, but that doesn't mean I'm useless. It also doesn't mean that I'm 'not the person I should be to them'. These are just stories that I am telling myself because I feel shit about myself. In this instance, I made mistakes, but rather than learn from them,

I have let the thoughts generated from them convince me that I'm a certain type of person. My mistakes haven't been a signpost as to what to do better next time, as they should be – instead, I have let them become a definition of me. All because my thoughts have gone unchecked and taken me down this path. And this path is one that leads me to make more poor decisions around my mental health because I think so little of myself. I will drink more alcohol and do even less to look after myself as my self-esteem hits the floor. And if I let these thoughts grow in my mind, they become my reality and turn into a long-lasting pattern. When I didn't have the awareness I do now, I would just sleepwalk into my next bad decision, thinking that's what life was like for me. But when I started to become aware of this, it was like a light switched on – I finally didn't have to believe these stories in my head. It was such a relief!

I can guess what you're going to ask next – 'If some thoughts are not real then how do I know what is a real thought and what isn't?' Well, that's a fair question because sometimes your thoughts are real. But the point here is to simply take the time to ask yourself. The important bit is found in the process rather than the answer. Because by questioning whether a thought is real, you create space between that thought and the potential bad action – space in which you can change your mind and react differently. You're not sleepwalking anymore.

Let's use my example above again. Rather than following on with this thought that I have let people down and I am useless, I stop and ask myself whether that is true. Immediately, I have paused the train of thought taking me towards a bad decision and have a chance of making a better one. Once I have acknowledged to myself that my feeling is not real, I then completely stop the train. I am therefore very likely to make a healthier decision in handling it.

Let me give you another example, which is slightly different – 'I think I have upset someone.' If I run with that thought unchecked, I can tell myself all sorts of stories about what type of person I am, what type of person they are and tie myself up in knots. And when I do that, I am very likely to make poor decisions. On the other hand, if I recognise that my thought might not be real and take time to check it by, for example, asking the person, then I can stop the negative thoughts spiralling. So, the solution in this example is not necessarily about whether I did upset someone, it is about giving myself some space to interrogate the thought. When I do that then I have a much better chance of dealing with it in a healthy way.

There is a layer to this that is even deeper. The chain that I have described so far starts with a feeling. But I have learned that I can also take time to analyse where that initial feeling comes from. I'll give you another example based on the situations above: 'I feel disliked because one of my old friends doesn't greet me as enthusiastically, and as a result, I decide to blank him going forward because I don't want him to do that to me again.' This example starts with me feeling disliked and hating the rejection that I am perceiving. Now, I can just accept that's how I feel or I can take a moment to ask myself why I am feeling like that. It's actually a great general question – why do I hate a potential rejection so much? We can all be hurt by rejection, but why do I react to it so strongly? Sometimes it's really hard to analyse things like this, but if we want to stop it taking control of us then it is crucial to try.

Why do I *have* to be liked?

Why am I so special that no one can dislike me?

When I face these uncomfortable questions head on I begin to see that the answer is because I am not feeling that great about myself. The whole thing is not about the other person's reaction to me, or my interpretation of it; it's about what's going on inside my own head. If my self-esteem is low then I start subconsciously looking for affirmation from other people. I want to be liked because it gives me that reassurance that I'm alright, that I'm a decent person. As, at that moment in time, I'm not feeling it myself. Meanwhile, the thought that I am being rejected is confirmation to me that I'm not a good person. That little voice in my head says, 'See? I told you that you were a dick.'

The solution to this is recognising that I need to address

my self-esteem. The other person might not like me or might have just had a lot of things on their mind that day, but by sulking and blanking them going forward, I'm not doing anything to make the situation better. By doing that I'm focusing on them and not on me. But if I can see that initial feeling for what it was – a symptom of my low self-esteem – then I can go away and work on that.

I know that when my self-esteem is shot it's because I haven't been practising healthy habits recently. This means that I won't have been keeping up with promises to myself and other people, and I will see that I am letting people down. The time when I let my sister down at the Ashes cricket at Headingley is a perfect illustration of this. My self-esteem was at an all-time low then and my actions were only compounding it. To get out of it, I needed to stop focusing on other people and get honest with myself.

I also needed to stop feeling sorry for myself – which feels like a subtle thread throughout this chapter. It's easy to do but does nothing to help. If ever the question 'Why me?' pops into your head while you're feeling sorry for yourself then immediately follow it with this question: 'Why not me?' I remind myself of this all the time. What makes me so special that I shouldn't have to experience difficult things in my life? Nothing. We all have challenges in our lives, and by avoiding a 'pity party' we live in the solution rather than the problem.

Take a moment now to consider when similar situations might have happened to you, maybe even today.

Did a feeling become so powerful that it consumed you or dictated your next actions?

Were the actions that followed ones that you're not particularly proud of now?

It could have just been a few sharp words with someone at work or a way you reacted to something your boyfriend or girlfriend did. Ask yourself where that initial feeling came from and what thought it produced before you took the action. Getting into the habit of investigating what lies behind certain feelings can be game-changing, giving us a chance in the future to alter the proceeding thought and finally the action. By doing this, we can stop self-destructive patterns of behaviour and protect our mental health.

One of the hardest things to handle with your mental health is feeling completely out of control. We feel like our minds have been taken over by crazy things we call anxiety and depression, and we can't shift them. It's horrible and very real. A black cloud swamps us like fog and we get lost in it. As true as this all is, what I have tried to show you in this chapter is that there are things within our power that we can do to help. It requires honesty and an acceptance of our personal responsibility on this journey, but we can do it!

Use this chapter to reflect back on your self-destructive patterns of behaviour and how honest you truly are with yourself. When you have done this then start to raise your self-awareness around your feelings and thoughts during those patterns. You will probably have to do this in real time and you won't always get it right, but that's part of being human. By simply attempting to challenge where feelings have come from and whether the thoughts that follow them are real you are already WINNING. Take it step by step, be as consistent as you can be, and you will slowly start to change how your mind works and prevent yourself from sliding into patterns that ultimately harm your mental health.

The ability to have greater self-awareness in our lives helps us so much. In the next chapter, I am going to be specific about this and how you can use certain aspects of self-awareness as tools in your day-to-day routines. Poor mental health can feel like it disempowers us, and these tools are going to bring some power back into our hands!

WHY NOT ME?

The tools that I now have to help me manage my mental health and sort out problems as they arise come from three particular areas of self-awareness. Having a good grasp of these has been so crucial for me. They will give you a far better chance of creating positivity in your life through healthy habits and actions. This then gives you a strong base that allows you to handle challenges or shifts that might arise with your mental health. Remember, it is all a compounding effect, so let's make that a positive one.

Here are three main areas of self-awareness that I have had to learn about to improve how I feel about myself and how I relate positively to the world around me:

Gratitude

I am a lucky man. I have been blessed with a body that allows me to achieve extraordinary physical feats, so much so that I have won medals in every major gymnastics tournament in the world. I am also blessed with an incredibly resilient and creative mind that has helped me build businesses outside of the gym. Finally, I am blessed to be surrounded by some amazing people, none more so that my family. My ma and pa gave me a sense of freedom and adventure as a child, encouraging me to reach for the stars and know that nothing is impossible, while my little sis, Joanna, is simply one of the best people you could ever meet. Like I said, I am a lucky man; and yet . . . in the blink of an eye, I can forget all of that.

Let me give you a fairly recent example. I have already talked you through why my experience on *Dancing on Ice* was so massive for me. It truly came at the perfect time, when I was at a crossroads in my life. I needed to compete again to scratch that itch but I also needed to discover who I was when it was all over. I know that I will look back on it in years to come and realise how lucky I was to have had that opportunity. And yet, with two or three weeks to go of the show, I started to resent it all. I found the schedule annoying, and mentally I started to get into a place where I wanted it all to be over. I was turning up late for filming and training, and generally complaining a lot about it. People were knocking on my door to wake me up to go to practice more times than they should have needed to. *Dancing on Ice* was incredibly positive for me and I still got into a headspace that meant I forgot all about that and only saw the negatives. Genuinely . . . what the fuck?! How could I get myself to a place where I felt like that?

As I look back on it, I'm a bit shocked. The entire show was really long and demanding, so I can understand why I was so tired, but the leap from loving it to resenting it is one that puzzles me. You might ask how this fits into how I manage my mental health. We can all be grumpy at times, right? Is it that big a deal in this context? Well, yeah, it is. If I lose perspective for my gratitude in life then it directly affects my mental health. When this happens, I don't think in a positive way and life begins to feel really heavy.

The good news is that I have found simple ways to practise gratitude on a daily basis and avoid getting into this headspace. I now know that I need to remind myself to do this regularly or I can easily slip back to being that ungrateful nobhead! Ha-ha! Later in this book, I am going to talk about daily routines in more depth, but the reality is that good habits require discipline and there is no getting around that. Here are the tips I want to share with you that will help you to practise gratitude:

1. Gratitude lists

An oldie but a goodie! Every day, write down five things you feel grateful for. I'm not having it if you tell me there's nothing for you to be grateful for. Everyone has something to feel grateful for in a day! Damn it, we are lucky to be alive and have a crack at life for starters. I find that first thing in the morning is best for me to write my list, but last thing at night also works. Having said that, it will do you no harm to write a gratitude list at any time in the day. Examples of things you can feel grateful for are people or animals in your life, a skill you have, a lesson you have learned, your health, nature or even simply things that make you laugh. The important bit is that you take a moment to consider gratitude rather than just letting it all slip by you.

2. See everything as an opportunity to grow

This means that when you are faced with situations that you don't immediately like, view them through the lens of an opportunity rather than a hassle. By doing this, you will then feel grateful for those challenges because they give you a chance to improve yourself. You don't learn patience without having to wait; you don't learn to be brave without being scared and you don't learn to be successful without failure. Every challenge is an opportunity to grow beyond it; we just need to embrace it. I am going to talk about this more later . . .

3. Get outside

If I feel myself sliding into a place of feeling grumpy with the world, I get outside and spend time with nature – and the bigger the look at nature, the better! Realistically, if my head is stuck in my phone then I have no chance of getting some perspective back. But if I go for a long walk with my ma along the Leeds and Liverpool canal then it reminds me of the big wide world out there and how beautiful it is. It reminds me how small my worries can be and how lucky I feel to be able to experience it all.

4. Think of others

There are always people worse off than you. Always. As I feel myself getting sucked into my own head and believing that my issues are bigger than anyone else, I step back and think of other people with far bigger problems than mine. I cringe at me being the guy complaining about the training schedule for a reality television show when there are countless people who would do anything for that opportunity.

Self

I believe that this word 'self' is really misunderstood by people. It's definitely something that took me a long while to get my head around. I had always just presumed that self was associated with 'selfish'; as in, it was just about when I or someone else was doing something for their own benefit, even at the sacrifice of someone else's. Well, it's more subtle than that. We can all be selfish sometimes. But understanding why and how that is happening is really important. Even if it doesn't always feel that comfortable. Let me attach this 'self' to three other words to show you how it can have different implications: 1) Self-serving, 2) Self-absorbed and 3) Self-care.

1. Self-serving

This quite literally means what it says – it is something you do that serves your*self*. So, it is an act that is in my best interests rather than anyone else's. Sometimes this is simple and totally fine. For example, training in the gym. My training is to make me stronger and better and is therefore self-serving. But there is also a different way to look at this. If we do a kind act for someone else you would think it is to serve them, not you. But is it always? How often have you done a nice thing for someone but hidden underneath the gesture is a desire to be recognised for it? Yeah, it's kind, but it's not coming from an entirely pure place. Secretly, you are expecting to get something out of it too. Now ask yourself whether you have ever felt disappointed when someone hasn't recognised your kindness. Don't get me wrong, this doesn't make you a bad person, but it is still something we have to recognise.

During Covid, I did a fundraising effort for NHS nurses on YouTube. I used my platform to raise money for what most people would agree is a really good cause. But was it completely for them? If I'm honest, I know that I got recognition from it and I got more views on that video. I raised some decent cash for a cause I cared about, but there was definitely a self-serving element to it. You see, the question to ask myself in that situation was what was I doing for the NHS nurses in the quiet when no one could see me? When there was nothing coming back to me other than a sense that I was doing a good thing?

Well, what I know today is that if my life is dominated by too many self-serving acts then everything becomes a transaction for me – 'I'll do this for you, if you do this for me.' When everything is some sort of exchange and there are no pure intentions that isn't healthy for me – or anyone. Everything gets complicated and fake. I lose track of who I am and the person I want to be. I lose the purity of my relationships and start to get disappointed with so much because, deep down, I am looking for something in return for everything I do. It's a dangerous mindset to be in because it doesn't make me feel good about who I am. My self-esteem drops, my sense of purpose drops and my view of the world gets dark and narrow. It's not who or where I want to be.

So, I challenge you now to ask yourself how many of your actions in a day, a week, a month or a year are actually self-serving? Is there an imbalance to this in your overall living? You don't have to tell anyone, but you do have to get really honest with yourself. Go on, do it right now.

2. Self-absorbed

God, this has been a massive learning curve for me! The thing is that all elite athletes are self-absorbed – we have to be! I don't know any top athlete in the world who isn't completely obsessed with what's going on for them over anyone else. The reason for this is simple – when I competed in an Olympic final in the horizontal bar, I was performing in front of millions of people under the most intense pressure imaginable. And I wasn't just parking my car! I was throwing myself around a metal bar at high speed trying to perform skills that have taken years to master. In order to get to that level of performance, you have to be completely self-absorbed. You don't have time to consider other people's feelings when you need to focus your entire energy into what you're doing. It is why we athletes can be really difficult people to live with. It has to be our way or no way. Your girlfriend might want to go out for someone's birthday, but you want to train more or get to bed early, so she will either go on her own or neither of you go.

Of course, this is my experience as an elite athlete, but the reality is that we all have the ability to become self-absorbed. We can all get lost in believing that what is happening for us is the only thing that matters in the world. Unfortunately, when we do this too often then it can really affect our mental health. When I was an elite gymnast, everything was about me. My family and friends always put my needs ahead of theirs, and when I retired this all came crashing down on me. Suddenly I was a 'normal person' and I discovered that you can't live your life like that in the real world. Being self-absorbed was necessary, and therefore forgiven, in elite sport, but, in the outside world, it isolates you. It disconnects you from people because you show no interest, empathy or understanding with what they are doing. That girlfriend who was patient with your behaviour while you prepared for the Olympics is going to lose all that patience when you show no respect for what she wants in her life. We know that poor mental health isolates you, and if your lack of awareness around how self-absorbed you are makes this worse for you then you are at the start of a slippery slope.

So, again, can you think about your own behaviour in the last day, last week, last month or last year – how have you been self-absorbed? Have you taken time to think about the needs of people around you? Have you listened when they have needed to be heard? Have you placed someone else's interests over yours at certain times? As ever, be honest with yourself. I would suggest that you write everything down so you can look back over it again. It might not feel that great to do, but it will feel amazing when you confront this and make any changes you need to.

3. Self-care

When I think of the phrase 'self-care', I immediately think of back massages and foot rubs! It's like popping into my ma's hair salon at their house in Pudsey for a good chinwag and a trim. Well, again, it *is* that to some extent, but there are more layers to it. Self-care is essentially actions that we take to look after ourselves – they keep us healthy. So yes, this includes nutrition, exercise, sleep, chinwags and foot rubs, but what I want to explain to you is how to have a broader view on this.

Let's start from here: are there actions or relationships that you are in today which undermine your self-care? You might be reading this thinking that's ridiculous, but is it? Are there or have there been relationships or friendships in your life which have actually been quite toxic? I can definitely say yes to that. Do you feel like your work drags you down every day? Do you get talked into going on nights out that you really don't want to and later regret? Yeah, been there. Do you find yourself hanging out with so-called friends that make you feel shit about life afterwards? Maybe you get belittled around them or they spend the whole time talking badly of others? If you're answering yes to any of these then you're doing things that are not healthy for you – you're not practising self-care. It's mad that we do this because it means that we basically don't value ourselves enough to create boundaries to stay away from these sorts of things. We don't prioritise self-care over things that make us feel shit in life. Why would we do that?

Well, I have done them all and I know how I made that switch to step away from this. I mentally started to honour and respect the importance of self-care in its entirety. I stopped thinking about the subject as being a trip to the health spa and more about my day-to-day living. As soon as I changed my perspective on it, it became more important to me and I became more self-aware of whether I was doing things to keep me healthy or not. I'll give you a simple comparison in my life. When I was in my teens, I trained so hard in the gym that it didn't really matter what I ate. I wouldn't put on weight because I was burning so many calories in the gym and my metabolism was fast. But then British Gymnastics brought in a sports nutritionist for the first time, and I listened to her about why our diet was so important to help us recover better in order to train or compete well the next day. Suddenly I made a connection in my mind that what I ate was key to my performance and I paid far more attention to it. I began to respect my nutrition far more and, like flicking a switch, my attitude to it changed immediately. There is no difference here to what I am talking about with self-care. Shift your perspective on it and start recognising that it is crucial within our day-to-day living, not just when we treat ourselves to a foot rub!

Responsibility

It is incredibly important that we don't believe that the journey with our mental health is completely out of our control. There are daily actions and habits that we can choose to do that will have a positive compounding effect on our mental health. Personal responsibility has already been an important thread in this book, but I am going to give you a broader perspective on it. Responsibility for our mental health is about owning the fact that there are actions that we can choose to do to benefit us on this journey. However, there is another aspect to responsibility that I want you to embrace to improve your self-awareness. Responsibility is also about recognising *your* part in ANY situation. Let me give you three super-quick examples:

- You're late for work and someone is driving really slowly, so you start raging at them. Your anger is directed at them but whose responsibility is it? Yours, because you left too late.
- You've run out of money towards the end of the month and you start moaning that your job doesn't pay you well enough. You're annoyed at your work for the situation you're in but whose responsibility is it? Yours, because you didn't budget your money well enough over the month.

- Your friend, who is always late, is late again for your
  lunch meeting and you're fuming at him. Your
  annoyance is pointed straight at your friend but
  whose responsibility is it? Yours, because you know
  he's always late and you've allowed it to happen
  again.

These are pretty simple, everyday examples, but the same
principle applies when the stakes are higher too. For example,
in 2015 I competed in the European Games 2015 in Baku,
Azerbaijan. It was my first competition back after a wrist
injury. I'd needed to have cartilage repair surgery on it. This
was a full British Olympic Association event, which meant we
competed as Team GB. Essentially, it was like a mini-Olympic
Games. During the competition, I fell off the parallel bars,
the horizontal bar *and* the pommel. Unsurprisingly, I didn't
make any of the individual finals. This was almost unheard
of for me – particularly on the parallel bars and horizontal
bar. I felt a mixture of heartbreak and embarrassment. This
was the sort of competition I would expect myself to excel
in, but I flopped badly. With my feelings being so raw, I
could easily have slipped into blaming someone – my
coaches, the medical team or even the equipment. But the
truth is that I wasn't as well prepared as I would normally
be. A lot of this was out of my control because of my

rehabilitation from an injury in the run-up to the competition, but it was my responsibility to choose how to react to the situation: start blaming people or outside factors, or get an understanding of what level my preparation needed to be at in order to do well in major competitions. One option was a pit of shit and the other was a solution.

In my eyes, responsibility is about looking at every situation and seeing what *we* could have done better rather than pointing the finger at someone else. The 'Blame Game', where we choose to blame someone else for a situation rather than look at ourselves, is a bottomless pit of negativity. We don't find solutions because we are not truly looking at the problem, we are just choosing to blame so we stay stuck. Blaming feels like a quick fix, but it's not. This is not to say that on some occasions another person doesn't carry some responsibility for what has happened, but the point is that by focusing all your energy on blaming them, you won't find a way out of it. Have you ever met a person who is constantly blaming other people and is a pleasure to be around? No. Do those sorts of people ever look like they are moving forward and enjoying life? No. We don't need to live our lives like that. Adopting an attitude of taking responsibility for any situation by looking at what we could have done better or what we can do better going forward means we live in solutions and not problems. I think of it as living in the sunshine rather than living in the drizzle!

I am fortunate to have played a part in building some really cool companies, no more so than Nile Wilson Gymnastics. Our team is constantly faced with problems or things that are not going as well as we would hope. If we had an attitude of blaming others, we would never find our way through these challenges and it would be a horrible place to work for everyone. Instead, we live in solutions but taking personal responsibility.

So there you have it. Reminding myself to be grateful, knowing when a behaviour is self-serving, self-absorbed or not aligned with my self-care, and taking responsibility for things that happen in my life are the three key tools of self-awareness that have made a huge difference to me. Of course, it's an ongoing, probably life-long (I'll let you know!) process, and it's not like I get it bang on all the time. But just knowing that I need to try and following through with that is so important so as not to get back on that slide down into a dark place. These things really do work.

As you will have figured out by now, so much of taking ownership of and improving your mental health is about making these good choices. So, in the next chapter, I'm going to show you how you can make it easier for yourself by creating structure in your life. For someone who can be as unstructured as me, this was a big lesson!

WHAT HOLDS ME UP IN THE WORLD

What is that old saying about only appreciating stuff when you've lost it? Ah yeah, that's it, 'You never know what you've got till it's gone.' Well, that was very much my experience with structure in my life.

After it was clear that my neck injury would never repair to the point where I could compete at the highest level, I had to retire from gymnastics. But what I didn't realise at the time was how many things I would lose at that point. I lost the opportunity to compete in the biggest arenas in front of thousands of people. I lost the status of being a professional gymnast. I lost a sense of purpose in my life. I lost that joy in mastering a new gymnastics skill. I lost a clear pathway to staying physically fit. So yeah, I lost a lot, but one thing that I unknowingly lost turned out, surprisingly, to be the biggest thing: structure.

Up to that point, I never realised how structured my life was as a professional athlete and, more importantly, how much I desperately needed it to be. I still feel really weird saying that because anyone who knows me, knows that I have always been pretty disorganised and don't always pay much attention to detail. (I daren't tell you the story about how I didn't open my post for six months and ended up with a driving ban!) And yet, I was (and am) a person who needs structure in my life, even though I can appear to others as being someone who lives life quite loosely.

Part of the reason why I didn't think I needed it actually came from a misunderstanding of what structure actually is. Structure is different to routine. They are very closely linked but they are separate things to consider. I want you to start to think of structure as being the very foundation of how you live your life, whereas routine is about regular habits that you develop within structure. Structure is the thing that pulls together and underpins what you are dedicating time and energy to in your life. I also know that every single one of us needs structure in order to protect our mental well-being, though not all of us are so into routines. Before we continue, take a moment now to think about whether you consider yourself to be someone who lives their life with or without structure.

When I was a gymnast, the structure that underpinned my life was built around four key things:

1. Training/competing.
2. Creating content for YouTube and other platforms.
3. Spending time with my family.
4. Spending time with my friends.

I'm not saying that was all I did with my life but, essentially, everything was based around these four pillars. Out of the four, training was easily the biggest. It's the one I dedicated the most amount of time to and it happened at set times. Whether I was training once or twice a day, training started and finished at the same time, every time. I knew exactly what I was meant to be doing. Everything else, including eating and sleeping, fitted around my training. Training was so much a part of my life that I didn't even consider it being something *in* my life, rather it *was* my life. If someone asked me what I was doing on a given day, week or month, my first thought would be training.

When I retired, I lost that enormous pillar of training and it felt like a huge hole had opened up in my life. Yes, I still had the other three, but they were fundamentally based around my training. Without me really realising it, I had organisation in my life through this structure. When training disappeared, that time needed to be filled, and that was the start of a lot of issues for me. I filled that time with drinking or gambling to distract myself, or else I would be left at home to ruminate on my own with my thoughts, which I found so hard and would lead to eventually drinking or visiting the casino. As you'll remember, being left alone with my thoughts was a really dangerous place for me. Before I started to put into practise the lessons in this book, I found that 'quiet' very uncomfortable – unbearable, in fact – because I had to sit still with myself, which, I now realise, I had always tried to avoid.

I did try to use this extra time I had on my hands to create more content for my online platforms, but it wasn't sustainable. I used to train for between 20 and 30 hours a week, and there was no way that I needed that amount of time for content. I also realised that I didn't have the passion to spend that amount of time on it. I enjoyed it and liked how it had previously fitted into my life, but it wasn't the main focus. So, there was still so much dead time in my life and everything felt unstable. I couldn't even hang around with some of my mates because they would be doing normal nine-to-fives.

The mad thing about all this is that when you're a full-time athlete, you always dream about the day when you can have loads of time to do other stuff – and then when it arrived, I was fucked! I wasn't ready for it. I made poor decisions during that dead time and would end up going to bed at 2 or 3am and then waking up at midday. It was really unhealthy. I started to take less care of my physical appearance and lost a lot of weight because all my muscle mass started to disappear, as I ate poorly and did little-to-no exercise. The compounding effect of it all meant that every day I was putting another brick onto the walls that would eventually close around me. It has taken me a long time to understand all this, and that when I started the training for *Dancing on Ice* it was why it felt so brilliant. Suddenly there was structure and purpose back in my life. All the ice-skating training slotted into the very place that my gymnastics training had been.

I believe that everyone can relate to my experience regardless of whether you are an athlete or not, because this isn't just about losing structure in your life, it is also about how your different pillars complement each other. In my case, I lost a huge pillar that I found hard to replace, but it was also about how it impacted the other three. For example, spending time with my family is everything to me, but that changed because suddenly I wasn't looking after myself properly and started to isolate myself. Even though family was a crucial pillar in my life, I got to a place where I avoided spending time with them. It was all so back-to-front. With more time available, you would think that I would have had more family time, but it was actually the opposite.

So, without any real thought, I was now losing two pillars. The same applied to producing online content. As my unhealthy life became more embedded, I started to lose all my discipline and motivation. Even though I had more time to create content, I now couldn't be arsed to do it. It was all so self-defeating. Having lost one major pillar in my life, all the others started to wobble and eventually collapse in on themselves.

It might be that you are already thinking about the pillars that exist in your life as you read about my experience. They could be things like your family, your friends, your physical health, your work, spending time in nature or a particular hobby or passion. What supports you, holds you up and makes you feel like you? I want you to take some time to think this through and write them down, as it's so important to understand what this means for you. To help you, try using these guidelines:

1. You should have a minimum of four pillars in your life.
2. Ask yourself if your pillars are all healthy for you.
3. Ask yourself if your pillars complement each other.
4. Ask yourself if one pillar dominates the others.

For most of us, working to earn a living is going to be a main pillar. Maybe you love your job and it's a big part of who you are, but even if you don't, it's still somewhere you have to be and something you spend a lot of your time doing. But also examine how that fits in with the other important aspects of your life. For those people who are extremely motivated to do well in their work, there will be times when it's going to dominate your life – but recognise that any structure cannot be held up by just one pillar. If your work begins to take away more and more of your time and focus from the other three then eventually that structure becomes unstable and collapses.

This very much applied to me while I was an elite gymnast. If my life only involved training and competition, and there was nothing else, then I would fall apart. I had a really early lesson in this when I went to the 2012 European Junior Championships in Montpellier, France, when I was 16 years old. It wasn't the Olympic Games but it was a big moment in my gymnastics career, and it turned out to be a pivotal one. Our intensity around winning was like nothing else and we felt under enormous pressure. It was all about the outcome.

We won the team competition, which was what all the focus was on. I won silver in the all-around, behind my teammate Frank Baines, and also made the high bar final. Delivering in my first major competition was a big step forward for me. And yet, although the results were what everyone wanted, I just didn't enjoy it at all because the pressure on the outcomes was suffocating. I learned that I didn't react well to that environment and the first signs of an eating disorder appeared. I became obsessed with losing weight under the belief that the lighter I was, the better I would be.

In the three months running up to these championships, I lost nearly 10kg. From 61kg to 52kg, it was total madness. I developed really bad issues with binge eating. Some people think that binge eating is just someone overindulging, but I can tell you from personal experience that it is much more than that and a serious mental health issue. I would be extremely disciplined with my eating for a period of time, not touching anything that I believed would make me put on weight. This was, I hope you can see, far from rational thinking. So I would barely eat but, eventually, the focus on what I should and should not eat would overwhelm me and I would blow. Once that happened, I was out of control. Two or three hours could go by without me really knowing what had happened. This was not me eating a bit too much chocolate or an extra bowl of ice cream; I kept eating more and more and more, four or five times the amount I needed, until my stomach was uncomfortably full. Sometimes, I didn't stop until 3am. It was horrible. Then shame and massive guilt would hit me. 'Why have I done this?' 'How did this happen?'

It would have a hugely negative impact on the following few days, as I convinced myself that I had to solve the problem I had created by hardly eating at all while trying to train hard. And then again, the pressure cooker would be building up and bang – it would happen again. I'd be back in the vicious cycle. I was stuck in a trap that I couldn't get out of. It tortured me and it was all driven by this intense focus on winning that overrode any other need I had in my life. The impact that this had on my training was really significant. There were times when I was training with no nutrition inside me, and times when I was trying to punish myself after a huge binge by training insanely hard. The likelihood of me getting injured was far higher and the quality of my training became really poor. Even though I was training on these days to improve my physical condition, the effect of my terrible relationship with food meant the opposite was happening. All of this continuously played on my mind and affected my mental health negatively. In the end, it took me being honest about this issue to my family and receiving help to gradually pull myself out of that horrible cycle.

If I take this back to the pillars that make up the structure in our lives, one of the underlying causes was that, at that moment, my gymnastics was far too dominant and it created real unhappiness for me. I need time in my life to appreciate other things, including time when I can laugh with my family and friends. It helps give me some perspective and balance to everything that I am doing.

Another important thing for me to reflect on here is that if everything is laser-focused on the result or the outcome then I am creating a very binary measurement on my life's happiness – win/good or lose/bad. It's too all-or-nothing. That doesn't work for me and I don't believe it works for anyone else. The structures cannot be held up by one thing alone without some sort of crash eventually. There needs to be an appreciation in your life for multiple pillars and how they all work together.

I do want to be clear on something, though. I believe that the idea of achieving perfect balance in life is impossible, especially if you are deeply passionate about something. I think that perfect balance is something that people spend far too much time mistakenly trying to achieve. The truth is that there are always going to be fluctuations in what takes up more time in your life. I wouldn't have become an Olympian if I had dedicated the same amount of time to my friends as I had gymnastics. Likewise, when you have a new baby, it will rightly dominate your time, as will exams or deadlines at work. Trying to achieve things or do the best you can in a certain situation sometimes requires a big time investment. Imbalance should be expected, and in certain periods there will be significantly more of it in your life, but if that is your constant state then there will be problems eventually. You will burn bright but not for long. So, even though perfect balance is unrealistic, you need to keep a gauge on how far out of balance you are at any one point.

If there is only one pillar in your life then it will be impossible to sustain good mental health.

Now that you've had a good think about the existing pillars in your life, I want to give you some suggestions on how to realign them, if that is required. The reason that I suggested four pillars to you is because I believe this is a healthy number. Any less and I think you're too close to a major imbalance happening, because it makes it more likely that one is more dominant than others. There's no harm in it being more than four, but that's how it is for me. To give you a sense of how this works in my life, these are mine now and why they are important to me:

1. Family and friends

I appreciate that not everyone has as close a family as us Wilsons, which is why I have included friends in this, but I do know that humans need humans. We need that connection with other people to feel safe and understood in the world. When I am head down, working like crazy on something, I struggle to see the overall perspective of what I am doing, and it's at times like this that I desperately need my family and friends. I'm pretty sure that the same will apply to you. How much time in a week do you spend with your family or very close friends? Do you consciously make time for them, even when you're busy? Do you have the opportunity to have open conversations with family or friends about how you are and how they are? If you don't then you should really have a think about it. For me, this is an absolute must in my life.

2. Work

I appreciate that there are people who are unable to work or who choose not to, but for the vast majority of us, we need to earn a living to pay our bills and live our lives. So this has to be a pillar we consider within this discussion. For some people, going to work is just something they have to do, while others will be fortunate enough that their work is also a passion that earns them money – my work is a mixture of the two. It comes in the form of creating content for my online businesses, working on television, working with brands and working to support my gymnastics clubs business. Some of it I adore and some of it creates the same mundane feeling that many people feel around their work. The important point to consider is how your work complements everything else in your life. Does your work come at the consistent detriment to other pillars in your life, and how does that make you feel? Are there times in your life when your work dominates everything but then you are able to pull it back to some relative balance? Do you love your work or do you love working? If you truly love your work then it is likely to be a passion of sorts for you and then potentially crosses over into two pillars in your life. Or if you simply love working and feeling purposeful in this area, then it would be really important to keep this in a healthy balance with the other pillars in your life. I want you to take some time to really consider how your work pillar sits and affects the overall structure of your life.

3. Passion

This has been a huge one for me to understand and develop. You see, for me, gymnastics was both my work and my passion. I was fortunate to be paid when I was part of the elite gymnastics programme in the United Kingdom, but the truth is that I would have done it for free if I could afford it. I was in love with the art we could create in the gym and the challenge of having to master incredibly difficult skills. And, as I've mentioned before, I loved to perform in front of people. It is why I was left with such a huge hole to fill when I retired. I needed to rediscover what I was passionate about, but before I did that, I filled that hole with unhealthy things like booze and gambling because I didn't know what else to do.

It's taken me time but I've found that it is golf for me! I bloody LOVE golf. I love the challenge of trying to master it, and I get to be outside with my pa and my friends – it's honestly amazing. Golf will feature in every single one of my weeks if I can manage it. So, what are you doing in your week that feels like a passion? Following on from the point above, your work can be a passion of yours, but I would like you to consider something else in your life for this section. It could be something you do on your own or with friends. It could be described as your hobby. Are you making time for this each week, even when you're busy? If you're not then I really think you should!

4. Self-Development

This is going to be a pretty broad pillar because within self-development I am going to include all physical and mental wellbeing. So this includes going to the gym, meditating, reading or taking a course to help you develop yourself in some way, among lots of other possible things. The point is that as humans, we need to keep growing to feel happy and alive. When we feel stuck is when we start to struggle. Throughout my life, the periods when my mental health has been at its best have been when I've been actively trying to develop myself by learning a new skill in or out the gym; listening to podcasts that I can learn from; educating myself with information I didn't know within my businesses and trying to be as healthy as I can physically be. So, this is a pillar that relates to anything that moves you forward as a person. Are you doing this right now? Are you actively looking to grow as a person in one way or another? Are you dedicating time each week for your self-development? Even when you're busy? I truly believe that this is a vital pillar and one that people sadly overlook sometimes.

I believe that these four pillars represent a solid structure for anyone, but others could be things such as charity, religion, financial independence or achieving milestones. We cannot ignore that most of us will need to work, and there are benefits to being productive on this front. Work gives us purpose, direction and, of course, money, but we need more than that in our lives.

Your pillars can change over time and, like I've said, they will fluctuate in dominance over each other depending on what's going on in your life. Don't waste time trying to achieve perfect balance, it's impossible, but keep a handle on whether one pillar is collapsing the others. Without an awareness of what your pillars are, how they fit together and how they create structure in your life, then you are left rudderless.

Before I lost competitive gymnastics as a huge structure in my life, I wasn't aware of how dependant I was on it. I had been doing gymnastics since I was four years old, and all my teenage and adult years were dominated by the sport. I didn't realise it, but gymnastics was a focal point for the entire structure of my life. The sport was even more important to me than I thought. Structure gives me a baseline to always go back to if I feel a bit lost or uneasy with life. The sorts of questions it draws me back to are, 'Am I making some time for *all* my pillars at the moment?', 'Is one pillar suffocating the others?', or, 'Are all my current pillars creating healthy outcomes for me?' Just simply taking time to ask yourself these questions is a win in itself. When I do it, it pauses me in life rather than allowing me to sleepwalk into a difficult place. Structure is different to understanding your daily habits, but they are aligned and this is what we are going to look at next. I would argue that without a clear structure in your life then healthy daily habits are impossible.

I hope you can see that with each chapter, I am encouraging you to learn more about yourself – because the answers to everything lie within. It is so tempting to always place mental health issues as something external that is happening *to* you. The real solutions to how we maintain healthy mental wellbeing start inside of us.

Greater self-awareness equals greater solutions.

EVERY DAMN DAY

When my depression and anxiety peaked in 2019, and my drinking and gambling were out of control, minutes became hours, hours became days and days became weeks. Everything was blurred into one and I just lost so much time of my life. I would stay up until 3 or 4am, either unable to sleep or messing around while drunk. The next day, I wouldn't wake up until after midday and then it was with the darkest feeling of dread. I knew there was a long list of things that I was meant to be doing and an even longer list of people that I felt I was letting down. I was a mess. However, nothing could shift the suffocating feeling of fear I had about the world in front of me.

My brain wouldn't shut up. I was fixated on what had happened and what might happen, never being able to enjoy where I was. I didn't want to talk to anyone. I didn't want to see anyone. All I wanted to do was curl up, cry and hope the day would be over quickly. And the weird thing was that

99

the day would be over relatively quickly. I might get out of bed at 2pm, and if it was winter, it would start getting dark in two or three hours. So I would get my wish and the day would be gone, and I would continue the same routine of not going to bed at a normal time, drinking and trying to escape the reality of the hole I'd got myself into. Back then, *this* was my daily routine, and I became chained to it because I couldn't see a way of getting out of it. In a really fucked up way, I was learning the power of your daily habits – it was just that those with all the power were unhealthy ones.

I'm not an organised or particularly detail-driven person. I go with the flow and am very much a 'feel' person, but, despite that, I have learned to understand the importance of daily habits. A good daily routine or set of habits doesn't make me an uber-organised person (although my manager, Luke, wishes it did!), but it definitely makes me a better version of myself.

There has been a lot said about the benefits of good daily habits, it is all over social media, but this chapter is very much about what works for me. I might not include some things that others swear by, but that's because those things aren't that important for me. This is as real as it gets, and my advice is based off that. I also know that how I fit my good daily habits into my day is very different to other people. I like to keep it as simple as I can, so that I can repeat it as much as possible. I'm not trying to be superhuman and I'm not going to be preaching to you about waking up at 5am, because I don't! Daily routines don't need to be a series of radically difficult tasks that some people proudly show on social media. I find meditation difficult and my routine doesn't even start at the same time every day! But, in my eyes, none of that matters, because it's about finding out what works for *you*. So, in that spirit, please take in what I describe to you about what I do but go on an adventure to see what works for you. There might be things I do that don't exactly work for you, and that's OK. All of us need healthy daily habits in our lives, but they don't all have to be exactly the same or be done at the same time.

I don't want this to look like a textbook or anything, but in the spirit of explaining what works for me, I think it's helpful to go over the main aspects of my daily routine so you can take any inspiration you want for creating your own.

Sleep

Whatever way we top and tail this, sleep is *so* important. When I was at my unhealthiest, it is no coincidence that my sleeping habits were at their worst. And sleep was a vital part of my recovery in between training sessions as a gymnast. During the last two years of my gymnastics career, I stopped taking any supplements that were meant to boost my recovery because I was so worried about accidently taking a banned substance in a supplement and failing a drugs tests. So I relied solely on sleep and it worked. When I slept well, my body recovered fantastically and I didn't need any additional help from a supplement.

I took my sleep super seriously and read up on it as much as I possibly could. One of the biggest things I learned was to wake up at the end of a sleep cycle, which happens every 90 minutes. This meant that I would always try to sleep for six hours, seven and a half hours or nine hours a night. The golden number for me was and still is nine hours. That may seem a lot to people, but through trial and error as an athlete, I worked out that nine hours' sleep is just perfect for me. If I consistently have that for a period of time then I feel mentally and physically incredible. Also, it may sound a bit pretentious, but I've invested money and thought into my bed! We spend a third of our lives in a bed so I wanted mine to be right for me. I have spent money on specific-thread cotton sheets, made the room completely dark with black-out blinds, controlled the temperature to keep it cool in there, and I have the correct pillows to support my neck.

Having said all this, though, I am not some sort of perfect sleep angel. I still sometimes stay up way too late and, like I said, I am certainly not a member of the 5am club! But I do respect the need for quality sleep, and getting to sleep before midnight is important to me now. We all have slightly different sleeping habits – for example, my sister wakes up at 6am every day – but the important bit is that we are getting seven to nine hours' sleep a night. I know that when I am tired, I am at my most vulnerable. If that happens too often then I go from vulnerable to being in trouble.

You can start your day whenever you want

I need to explain this one! While focusing on a daily routine, I think a lot of people get wrongly hung up on when to start and end their day. This might sound a bit weird, but hear me out. I constantly hear this line on social media, 'I start every day with . . .' and it infuriates me. By doing this, people are essentially placing expectation on exact periods of the day – i.e. in the mornings I do this, in the afternoon I do this, etc. But this kind of thinking is one of the things that seriously messed with my head when I was struggling. It reminds me of when I would weigh myself before a gymnastics training session. I remember looking at the number on the scales, and if it wasn't what I wanted, I would then get into the headspace of believing that I would have a bad session.

I can't tell you the number of times my head has told me that because I have fucked up one part of the day, I might as well fuck up the rest of it. Low self-esteem can cripple someone when expectations are placed on how a day should map itself out. So a HUGE learning for me was changing my perception of 'my day'. I realised that it doesn't have to be perfectly timetabled, perfectly planned; it doesn't need to be perfect, full stop. When life feels at its easiest for me, it flows – it doesn't need to be scheduled down to every millisecond. Some days I wake up on top of the world, and some days I wake up not feeling so great. Some days I start the day in the best possible way, and other days I *really* don't. But I don't believe that any of that should determine whether I have a good day or a bad day.

So, I would really like you to remember this: **you can start or re-start your day whenever you want**. If you get to 11am and it has been a total shit show up to that point then don't panic or write off the day because it hasn't been 'perfect' – just start again. Go through the steps that you know will give you the best chance of getting yourself in the best possible frame of mind and go again. If it turns out to be a real shit day, then you can do this as many times as you like. Don't get caught believing that your day should follow some exact pattern or schedule in order to be a good one. Life is just not that simple, and if your self-esteem is a bit rocky and you're feeling vulnerable then that pressure is just not helpful to you.

Take some time

I have tried over the years to get to what I perceive as 'good' at meditation, but the struggle has been real! My racing head just erupts into the most ridiculous explosion of thoughts as soon as I try to quieten it. It's actually pretty insane how noisy my head can get in the 'quiet'. Don't get me wrong, I have got so much better at it, but it is not something that has come easily to me. However, I did get a really good bit of advice once that changed my whole perspective on meditation. It was explained to me that there is no right and wrong in meditation – you can learn to master it, but actually the real success is simply in trying to do it. It took me some time to get my head around this. I eventually understood that I had been judging my meditation on how 'well' I did it rather than just appreciating the fact that the act of trying to meditate meant I was taking time out of my day to sit with myself, which was a success in itself.

If you are like me, then sitting with your own thoughts is something you probably really struggle with. The lesson that has come from this for me is that each day I need to take some time to sit with my myself, away from my phone or the television or any other type of electrical device. Just me on my own for 10–15 minutes. Yes, this could be called meditation, but it doesn't have to be. Call it something else if you prefer. In all honesty, it is more often just me sitting with a coffee on my balcony and listening to the world starting its day. And I don't need to judge 'how it went', there is no right or wrong to it. The win is just in doing it, because those minutes are crucial, as rather than rushing into the day without any real thought, I'm giving myself some time to centre myself, to calm myself, and remember who I am and who I want to be in this world. I promise, just ten minutes of that can be so precious within your day.

Cold start

I either have a cold shower or an ice bath every day, but ideally a bath. I just think it's fucking brilliant. Regardless of the science, I love the fact that it's so difficult to do. It's uncomfortable but it forces you to be super present when you're in there because basically you're freezing your bollocks off! This links with the point above about having some time to yourself to start a day through meditation or silent thought over a coffee. An ice shower or bath is another version of this because you have 60, 90 or 120 seconds, or whatever you can achieve, in which you are completely focused on your body. There is also the additional element of feeling like you have achieved something every time you do it!

Spirituality

This section title might have made a few of you jump! To be fair, it would have done the same to me a few years back. I need to explain this well because arguably it is the most important part of my daily habits. When I say spirituality, I don't mean any sort of religious god – not that there is anything wrong with that at all. What I mean is an understanding or appreciation on a daily basis that I am not in control of every outcome in the world. I know that sounds a bit mad, but I have learned over the years that my anxiety is chained to my head's ability to hyperfocus on outcomes. Outcomes of the past and possible outcomes in the future. In other words, when my anxiety is crippling me, I can't get past thinking about things that have happened and things that might happen.

For example, if I have been rude to someone while drunk then that would sit in my head for days or even weeks. I would beat myself up about it because I'd imagine this whole story in my head about how much they hated me and what a terrible person I was, all without knowing anything about how that person was actually affected by it or thinking what I could do to simply resolve it. It was like my head would get stuck in the mud and I couldn't let it go, while my anxiety would swallow me up. I have realised that behind all this was an illusion in my head that everything in the world centred around me. Every outcome was somehow linked to what I had or hadn't done or would or wouldn't have done. Weirdly, it was all really self-obsessed.

The strange thing was that I didn't have this sort of anxiety around my gymnastics, where I could be much more pragmatic about what I needed to do. I would focus on turning up for training, doing my best and letting the process take its course. It would be a step-by-step way towards success, without getting caught up in what may or may not happen in results. And yet, in my day-to-day life, I have found this much harder to practise. My only relief from it has been faith. I remind myself *at least* once day that all I can ever do in any given situation is to be the best version of myself. If, in that moment, I am not a great version of myself then all I have to do is attempt to be the best I can be for the next moment. I have faith in the universe to sort things out as they should be, and my part in that is just to put my best foot forward at any given point in my life. The phrase I often use is, 'Just do the next right thing.' And that's it – trust the universe to sort all the outcomes as they are meant to be, while I keep doing the next right thing. It's as simple as that and all lies in faith. I have to practise this on a daily basis to keep my head from spinning out of control.

Exercise

There is no question in my mind that taking care of your physical wellbeing massively helps your mental wellbeing. I have been very lucky that exercise, mainly in the form of gymnastics, has been part of my life since I was four years old. I learned how important it was to me when I went through periods of being injured, with my neck injury being the worst. Being physically incapacitated in one form or another takes so much out of me mentally; I just don't feel the same person. And this is much more than just looking good with a top off. Exercise is a form of self-care, release, peace, space, excitement, challenge, purpose and adventure that I find hard to replicate in so many other things. The correlation between not exercising regularly and my mental health being poor is obvious and inescapable. This is why exercise has to be a non-negotiable within my week.

I have highlighted five important areas for me within my day, but there are many more that could work well for you, including nutrition, prayer, reading, etc. I don't discount any of those things, but I would just be lying if I told you that they were things that I did on a daily basis. The question now is how does this all fit within a normal day for me. As I've said, I don't love the concept of imposing a strict formula on every day. I understand why people do this, but you are then chained to that routine, whether you think it's working well or not. I like to look at my day as being something much more fluid and changeable – so long as it includes the key things I have talked you through.

For example, taking some time to centre myself in my version of mediation is something that mainly happens in the mornings with a coffee. Why? Because it's normally the quietest time of the day to do that and it can start me off well. Likewise, I will often remind myself first thing in the morning of my faith in the universe and my job is just to do the next right thing, for exactly the same reasons. However, it doesn't have to be that way all the time. Sometimes, I rush out the door and forget to do those things, so I then find a quiet spot at the gym or a café to do exactly the same thing in the afternoon. Sometimes, I have those moments in my car at a traffic light. The crucial part for me is not when, but just that I do it.

I generally exercise in the afternoons, but not all the time. And exercise can take lots of different forms for me – gymnastics, weight training, running, golf or walking with my ma. Again, it is not when or how, it is just that it is a regular part of my day that is the important thing.

Although I take sleep very seriously and believe that good sleep is crucial to all of us, I am not locked in by exact bedtimes and wake ups. The key is that I am getting enough sleep for me. I like to be asleep before midnight so I get a full day the next day, but it doesn't always work out like that. I appreciate that I don't have a nine-to-five job, which would tie me to a time I needed to be up at, but my approach to sleep is much like my approach to the other important areas within my day – it's really important to me but it doesn't need to be dictated by a strict timetable.

My approach to daily habits is different to some of the other people that you might have seen on social media. But I just don't believe that it should be a box-ticking exercise or a competition with people around you. If it is then you won't be able to sustain it. You won't enjoy it and it will feel forced. In my opinion, a good day of habits is about *living* it rather than just *doing* it. It has to become part of who you are as a human being and feel right for you. As an example, for me to take time in each day to centre myself or remind myself of my faith in the universe, that can't be scheduled into an exact, fixed 15–30-minute slot – it has to be about much more than that. I have to feel these things sincerely and deeply so I can draw on them at any moment in my day. I can't just go through the motions. Likewise, if I am so regimented about the time I exercise each day and I miss that window for some reason, then I'm likely not going to be exercising. And I miss out an essential habit. Whereas, if I feel a need to exercise during my day then I will find the time. The whole thing is much more fluid and, in my mind, much healthier.

At the beginning of this chapter, I asked you to learn from my experience but also to go on an adventure of what you feel works for you. Take a moment to have a think about your daily habits.

Which would you categorise as 'good' and which as 'bad'?

What impact are they currently having on you?

Also, take some time now to think through what you would like your daily habits to be. You can schedule it if you want or you can just write down a list of things that you want to include in your day-to-day. Work out what's important to you, investigate why it feels so right for you, practise it on a daily basis and then eventually it becomes part of who you are.

I have briefly talked about exercise here, and now I want to give you a whole chapter on why it is so important to us and how it can help you to manage your mental health. And what I'm about to say might surprise you!

I CHOSE NOT TO

Ever heard the phrase, 'I'm just not motivated to exercise at the moment'? In this chapter, I am going to present to you different attitudes to exercise and motivation, and explain why they can be so beneficial to your mental health.

I guess it would seem pretty obvious that an ex-Olympian would want to tell everyone that exercise is important to have in their lives. After all, peak physical fitness has been part of my life since I was four. At the age of ten, I was training 24 hours a week and my life was school, gym, eat, sleep and repeat. I tell everyone that gymnasts are the closest thing to humans trying to make themselves fly, as we throw ourselves through the air at high speeds with multiple twists and turns. The truth is that what we can do with our bodies blows people's minds, which is why I think we are always one of the most watched sports during an Olympic Games.

What I love about gymnastics on the physical side is that through our training, our bodies become perfectly balanced. We are lifting our own body weight so our muscles become completely in tune with that. The positions that we have to put our bodies into result in a human physique that can be adaptable to anything. The muscle tissues that we create defy the opinion that you can't be powerful *and* flexible. We're the most flexible and strongest, relative to our weight, people on the planet. I have also never seen gymnasts pull a hamstring, yet footballers, cricketers, rugby players do it every week. I believe that gymnasts are the ultimate athletes. Granted, I am a little bit biased, but I think most people would find it hard to argue against that . . . !

I'm guessing, maybe wrongly, that you are expecting me to give you chapter and verse about setting yourself targets and training programmes, with motivational quotes alongside it as a bonus! Well, I'm not. Not because I don't think all of that can be helpful to some, but because I think we need to view exercise through a different lens, one which covers us all. Too often, I see exercise described as something that becomes too much, too intimidating for people. It's similar to how I talked in the last chapter about my belief that the concept of a daily routine can be so misplaced for many people. Exercise benefits our mental health enormously, but not by being something that means you compare yourself to others or expect things of you that are unrealistic. There can be something much more personal, authentic and healthy about exercise.

One of the greatest lessons that I personally had to learn about exercise is how much I attached my persona to my physical capabilities. I was 'Nile Wilson, an incredible athlete'! That was who I was – or, more accurately, who I believed I was. In my mind, my physical capabilities were inseparable from how good a person I was, how successful I was in life. But then what happened when I got injured and wasn't able to do the physical things I associated with my persona? I mentally fell off a cliff. In the two months after my neck surgery, I lost a stone in weight and I am not a big man. All my muscle wasted away due to inactivity, and with it my mental health withered away as well. I shared comparison photos on Instagram, and in the weight-loss photo I look like a little boy – it shocks people. My physical deterioration and my mental deterioration were intrinsically linked. As I recovered from this, I realised how misplaced my relationship with exercise was. If I wanted to find peace in retirement then I needed to change my perspective.

Have a think about what role exercise plays in your life. Maybe it doesn't at all. I am absolutely not here to shame you for that – or for anything. Although, of course, I'd love to encourage you to give it a try. Obviously, exercise is quite literally physical movement that increases our heart rate, muscle growth and overall health, but what else is it?

What does it feel like when you're doing it, whether in the gym, yoga studio, football pitch, squash court, on your bike or simply out on a walk? How would you describe that time of the day or week? Tap into how it feels emotionally for you. Ignore results, targets or goals – just simply how it makes you feel. Try writing these emotions down, because in doing so they will become much clearer to you. If you don't currently exercise, try to remember a time when you did do something physical and it felt good for you.

The best way I can describe exercise for me nowadays is that it is 'my time'. It's my time to be entirely present in what I am doing and get away from the stresses that life might have thrown up that day or week. Exercise is my escape. Sometimes I think of new ideas or a solution to a problem while exercising and I wonder why it has come to me then. Well, it's because all the noise of the world has died down in my mind and in the quiet comes new thoughts. It is a form of meditation for me. If my heart rate is going up with exercise, my nervous system is calming down at the same time. It's genuinely therapeutic for me in mind, body and soul. This is what I have discovered exercise should be about.

Now, please don't misunderstand me; I am a competitive beast and I love the challenge that physical training goals give me. This will never leave me; it's in my DNA – whether it is a certain weight to lift, a distance to run or a skill to be mastered. I have got really into jiu-jitsu in the last couple of years and it has all of these things. If you don't know what jiu-jitsu is, it is a self-defence martial art based on grappling and submission holds. It is ridiculously technical and so tiring! You try to use different holds and locks to get into a dominant position and submit your opponent. It is really difficult and I've been drawn to the challenge of it. Me and my mates, Luke and Ash, love having a go at it. It's a sport that makes you extremely present, a bit like how an ice bath does, but this time you have another man trying to beat you up. You're playing chess with your body and it's a really humbling experience. Starting the day by getting beaten up with jiu-jitsu and then having an ice bath is tough, but I love it. That's part of who I am and there is nothing wrong with that. I don't want you to think that I am suggesting exercise has to become this floaty, non-competitive, non-goal driven thing. I don't mean that at all. It can be as intense as you want it to be, but my point is that you don't have to see it as *only* about results, rather than the experience you get from it. If you get obsessed with results and targets, then you are getting attached to your physical capabilities, and if they go for any reason, with an injury, for example, then it can be a sharp fall. Embrace exercise, however intense or not it is, for what it is giving your entire body, including your mind. If you're injured and you can only walk rather than run, then that's still OK. If you have to change what you were meant to do because of schedule or circumstances, then embrace it. Appreciate the time it gives you away from the mad and hectic world. Enjoy the time to focus on yourself and the exercise you're doing, whatever that might be on the day. It is your time so love and appreciate it, rather than seeing it as something that deserves constant comparison, analysis and progress.

The other important point is not to worry about your ability levels or whether you are 'doing it well'; just embrace exercise as being time for yourself. I don't think you can go wrong with that mindset. Of course, there are other benefits to exercise, and if you love being part of a team then playing something like football or netball will be amazing for you. The camaraderie you get from being part of a team is something special, and it is no coincidence that I always performed at my best when I was competing in the team event in major gymnastics competitions – I absolutely loved that feeling of being part of something with my teammates. I'm not trying to diminish these sorts of things that come from different forms of exercise – just as much as I'm not saying you have to do this if you don't get the same rewards out of team sport that I do – but I just want to help you achieve a way of viewing it that is sustainable and embraces whatever level you are at. I totally understand that some of you might feel embarrassed or daunted to try a new form of exercise or to get back into exercising after a long time off it. But, remember what I have said above – just embrace exercise as being time for yourself. This is not about ability or results. You don't necessarily need to join a gym, club or team, just find time to go for a walk by yourself or with a friend. If you're feeling like this then that's a great start.

OK, now for motivation. I think I might also shock you in how I talk about this! Throughout my life, people have often said to me that I must have had incredible motivation to train as I did. They would comment that chasing an Olympic gold medal must have been an enormous motivation for me. Likewise, I often hear people who are not working at something, whether in the gym or at work or as a hobby, say things like, 'I'm struggling to find motivation.' And that's the issue – many people see motivation as something you need to find. They see it as something that you need to generate in order to do something difficult. I'm sorry to break it to you, but that's not true. This myth is based on two falsehoods that people believe in. The first one is that motivation is relatively permanent: i.e. I must have had a lot of motivation to train as I did. The second one is that motivation is something that you can continuously generate from within: i.e. a person can think of something on a particular day that will 'motivate' them to do something difficult that day. Unfortunately neither of these things are true. I'll explain why.

Nobody, and I mean nobody, has permanent or even

semi-permanent motivation. I have trained at an elite level for far more of my life than I haven't. I have literally lived it. I have also been surrounded by elite athletes from my sport and other sports, so I know what makes them tick. Motivation is nowhere near permanent. There are many more days than not when your mind and body says, 'I don't want to do this.' I rarely jumped out of bed and ran to the gym, no way. My body would be sore and the repetition of training would wear me down, and I would even be bored of it sometimes. I could remind myself that this was all about an Olympic gold medal, which is undoubtedly a huge thing, but even that wouldn't be enough on some days.

If you have been going to the gym every day for a month and you have started to physically look and feel better, then there will definitely be days when you wake up and feel like you can't be bothered. What keeps you going then? Your motivation has definitely waned so do you just reinvent or rephrase your 'motivation'? Of course not. Motivation ebbs and flows like the tide. Some days or weeks you feel pumped up and motivated to hell, and other days or weeks you simply don't. So if we recognise that we need exercise consistently in our lives then we have to start to see that motivation is not going to be the thing that keeps us doing it long term; it has to come from something else.

The second falsehood around motivation is that we can simply generate it or find it from somewhere when we need it. I cringe when I see some massive guy from a gym shouting into the camera, 'Go and find your motivation!' There will be times in your life when you will feel intensely motivated, and other times when you will feel nothing. Those intense moments will come from short bursts of emotion. They are great while they last, but if you rely on those then your success rate in doing what you need to do will fluctuate all the time. It's why people fall in and out of diets all the time. They start highly motivated to lose weight, but that motivation doesn't last forever so they stop doing it until they get motivated enough to try something new, and it goes on and on. The reality of that type of intense motivation is that it has often come from some sort of pain in your life – i.e. you now want to lose weight because it has reached a point that is unacceptable to you; you are short of money so the desperation to earn some more is very strong; you need to stop drinking because the doctor has told you that it will kill you. But is that really how we want to 'find' motivation? By reaching a point of pain that we are forced to change? If we want a life that is consistently healthy in body and mind then we can't get caught in this yo-yo trap where everything fluctuates so much. If we want exercise to be a consistent part of our lives then we need something else to focus us.

So, here we go . . . stop trying to 'find' motivation and replace that word with DISCIPLINE.

What kept me going to training day-in, day-out wasn't

motivation, it was discipline. And there is good news with this – discipline is available to all of us at any time that we want it! It is a choice that we can make or not make. There is no need to find it; it is quite simply a contract that we make with ourselves. Let me give you a simple example: you brush your teeth every day because you have made a sub-conscious contract with yourself to do it. You know it is healthy for your teeth and you like the feeling you get from it. You don't wake up and try to think of a motivation to brush your teeth – you do it as second nature because you have developed discipline for it from being a child and being reminded to do it on a daily basis, and then eventually making the choice to do it. Exercise is no different to that, whether at an elite level or more casually. Granted, exercise is more challenging than brushing your teeth, but if you have got into the habit of exercising every day or a certain number of days per week, you will know that it also feels like second nature to you.

My sister, Joanna, works harder than anyone I know – she's immense. She is up every morning at 6am and working almost immediately, as well as exercising and doing self-development stuff. I'm constantly inspired by her. When I ask why she does it every day, she says, 'It's just what I do.' She'll tell you her huge aims, but she backs it up with actions. She gets it done because she's so disciplined with it that it has become second nature to her. Like she says, it's just what she does.

Discipline is the cornerstone of developing healthy habits in your life, including exercising regularly. Like I have said, it is a choice that you can make at any time and you don't need to rely on motivation. But to make it happen, you need to acknowledge the personal responsibility involved. The next time you say, 'I could have exercised today but . . .' replace it immediately with, 'I chose not to exercise today because . . .'. Discipline is on us, no one else. It is a contract with yourself that you either honour or not, but it is your choice.

I want to let you into another secret involving motivation – discipline can actually help with creating motivation in your life, not the other way around. Discipline is what kept me going to training day-in, day-out. It drove me forward when I felt zero or little motivation, or was injured, or tired, or bored, or anything in the middle of all that. Trust me, there were many more 'off' days than days when I felt 100 per cent to smash training. Any athlete who tells you different is telling you porkies! When you are training at that level, you are almost never perfectly fit or healthy. There is always something you are recovering from or working around within your body. We simply can't push ourselves that hard without our bodies barking back at us, but that doesn't mean we can stop training. What keeps us going is . . . discipline. But then this magic thing happens. Discipline created consistency for me in my training, which made me stronger and more skilled at my sport. Relentlessly practising routines meant that I got fucking good at them! Constantly conditioning my body meant that I became super-humanly strong! And I could see that and I loved what it gave me. As I mastered a new routine on the high bar or parallel bars, my mind would immediately think, 'Right, what more can I do now?' I loved my progress and wanted more of it so I pushed for more. I would be immediately pressing my coaches to see what else we could do and what other skill we could add in to create more difficulty. Now *that* is motivation!

So, consider the process: discipline drove progress, progress drove enjoyment, and finally, enjoyment drove motivation.

Discipline can create motivation, but motivation is not long-term enough in nature to create your discipline. Understanding this is paramount to understanding how to consistently integrate exercise into your life, because it won't be driven by motivation; it will be driven by discipline. Discipline requires that you make a contract with yourself as to how you are going to keep or add exercise to your life. Accept and understand that it is a choice that falls under your personal responsibility. Remember, if the words, 'I could have' creep into your vocabulary then correct yourself immediately and say, 'I chose not to.'

I've been that person who says that I'm going to get up at seven and I get up at nine, who says I'm going to go to the gym this morning and then I don't go, who says I'm going to make my bed this morning and then doesn't do it. I think we all have. But when you actually do what you say you're going to do, with even the smallest tasks throughout your day, it gives you momentum and you feel proud of yourself, even for something so little.

Take some time now to consider where your attitude lies with regard to motivation.

Has anything in this chapter challenged your previous beliefs on it?

How do you think you can embrace some of the things I have said going forward in your life?

Developing this level of self-awareness is only going to benefit you, because the most important relationship we have in life is with ourselves. I am going to extend this point in the next chapter by looking at how we talk to ourselves through 'self-talk' and how that can affect us enormously.

ME VERSUS ME

The conversations we have with ourselves are the most important ones we have in our lives.

Did you know that experts estimate that the mind thinks between 60,000 and 80,000 thoughts a day? That's an average of 2,500 to 3,300 thoughts per hour. How many of your thoughts spark a conversation in your head? If you're like me, I bet you can't quantify that because it happens almost all the time.

The people close to us have a significant influence on our lives but we have a far more important relationship to think about, and that is with ourselves. How we talk to ourselves can enormously affect our self-esteem, our confidence and our overall attitude to life. In this chapter, I am going to explain this to you, challenge you to think about your current self-talk and what you can do to improve it.

How I handled my self-talk was a massive factor in my

success at the 2016 Rio Olympics. This was due to the relationship I had with a brilliant man called Michael Finnigan. I was first introduced to Michael by my dad. Dad used to work at Direct Line Group, one of the UK's largest insurance companies, and Michael had been brought in to run mindset sessions with some of the company's main leaders. The programme, conceived and written by Michael himself, was called 'Impossible to Inevitable', or 'i2i'. My dad was blown away by it and wanted me to meet Michael. We hit it off immediately and I loved everything that Michael was about.

The biggest thing Michael instilled in me was that I had the power to go out there and achieve greatness; whether it was in the gym or elsewhere – I could make the impossible inevitable. It was all about mindset. My mindset would drive my behaviours and my behaviours would drive my outcomes. Whenever I had time with Michael, all I could see ahead of me was opportunity. I fucking loved it!

In the four years running up to the Rio Olympics, I did an incredible amount of work with Michael over the language I used when I talked to myself. It sounds ridiculously simple, but the words 'I can do this' became an integral part of this. By the time I reached the Olympics, those words were so conditioned within me that they were a perfect representation of my whole-hearted belief in myself. I'll also add to this that in two years prior to the Olympics, every time I got in the shower I'd visualise nailing my routine. My dad has always said to me that the brain can't tell the difference between real and imagined. So, by the time the day of the Olympic final came in 2016, it had been the thousandth time that I'd visualised sticking my dismount and nailing my routine. I had a feeling of inevitability about it all.

On the day of my Olympic high bar final, all the finalists got a three-minute warm up on the bar, and I felt great after mine. All I said to myself throughout it was: 'I can do this.' Those words were as crucial to me as any physical warm up I could do. The intensity of the Olympic final was like nothing I had ever felt before and it's very difficult to describe. It's simply the biggest moment of your life. I had worked my entire life for this and there was no hiding from the fact that this was HUGE. I was about to be part of Olympic history in an arena with 20,000 people screaming in it and millions watching on television. There was no point in downplaying it, because the enormity of it all was inescapable. I just had to embrace it, and all I kept saying to myself was, 'I can do this.' Again and again. There were no inspirational words needed from a coach; it was just me and my belief in myself.

I was third up in the final, with Fabian Hambüchen going first and doing a brilliant routine, and then Epke Zonderland going second and falling. As I chalked up my hands and walked to the bars, time stood still. Fabian's brilliance and Epke's mistake had made no difference to me. This was about me, not them or anyone else in the final. It was just me versus me. Just before my coach lifted me on to the bars, I shouted one more time, 'I can do this!' I couldn't hear anything and I couldn't really feel anything – I was on autopilot. It was a blur. And then suddenly I was preparing for my release, I let go, I was in the air and my feet hit the ground. I stuck the dismount! As I straightened my legs, I felt this surge of emotion through my body as I screamed out loud and started laughing. I had nailed my routine on the biggest possible stage imaginable. 'I can do this' had become 'I have done this'.

That single moment in my life is the biggest example I can give you of the importance of self-talk. The Olympic final was so intense that it made conscious actions or decisions impossible. It really was just a blur, but, as I look back on it, I can see that I performed exactly as I had prepared. Physically, I was in exceptional condition; technically, I was performing a routine that I had done a million times and had truly mastered, and, crucially, mentally, I had complete and utter faith in myself. There was no doubt in my mind. 'I can do this' hadn't just been lame words; it had been a continual affirmation to myself that by the time I reached the Olympic final was flowing through my veins. I appreciate that an Olympic final isn't a day-to-day example to give you, but that's why I wanted to use it. If I can illustrate to you how it worked for me in a moment like that then imagine how we can use positive self-talk in our normal daily lives.

The first step in all of this is to simply recognise how often you speak to yourself and what that sounds like. Consider your self-talk now and write it down as you think through it.

Do you use language like 'I can do this' or is it more like 'I always make mistakes', 'I'm not good enough to do this', 'They hate me' or 'I am going to look stupid'?

Are there situations in your life that you find yourself in that feel completely overwhelming? If so, what sort of things do you tell yourself at that moment in time?

Imagine if I had been waiting to start my routine in the Olympic final and I was saying to myself, 'I'm not sure I can do this'. I would have carried that into the blur of my routine and who knows what would have happened. It's not dissimilar to having to make a big presentation at work and being crippled by self-doubt as you start.

There is one line that I used earlier that I really want you to remember. It has come from my work with Michael Finnigan: 'My mindset would drive my behaviours and my behaviours would drive my outcomes.' If you've still got your pen to hand, why not write it down?

Once we get honest about what our self-talk sounds like, we have a chance of changing it, if we need to, but the process is a gradual one. Remember, by the time I got to the Rio Olympics, I had been working with Michael Finnigan for four years. View it in the same compounding way that I have talked about managing our mental health throughout this book. A series of little positive changes compound on each other and eventually make a big positive difference. Changes can be subtle as well. I'm not expecting someone with very negative self-talk to suddenly walk around telling themselves they are superman or superwoman!

So, if going straight to 'I can do this!' would feel insincere or forced to you, consider this:

You can start by changing the words 'I can't do this' to 'I can't do this . . . yet'. Saying 'I can't do this' is creating an impression of a situation being permanent. 'I can't do this yet' means there is a process underway.

If you say to yourself 'I always make mistakes', you can replace this with 'I sometimes make mistakes while I'm learning'.

If this all feels really alien to you then it will feel uncomfortable doing this at first, but it does become easier.

If you're not sure how negative your self-talk is, ask yourself whether you would talk to someone you loved like that. Imagine yourself as a little boy or girl staring up at you – how would you talk to that younger version of you? What would you say to yourself as a child when you made a mistake? Would you be reassuring, encouraging, kind? How would you want you to feel? I'm sure you will feel compassion as you think about that, so start learning to use that sort of language and tone with yourself. Whenever you feel yourself drifting back to talking to yourself in a negative way then think about how you would talk to your younger self. The whole thing will require a lot of practice, but it is a process so give it time and be patient with yourself. No negative self-talk about self-talk!

Self-talk will always be enhanced by evidence. The words 'I can do this' kept affirming my belief in myself because I had done that Olympic final routine perfectly in practice and other competitions many times previously – it wasn't simply words. Sometimes this point is used in reverse to argue against using positive self-talk. If I were to ask someone not to use the words 'I can't do this', a response I could get back is, 'Well, I *can't* do this!' because the person is literally describing how they feel in that moment. Likewise, you could tell yourself a million times that you're the most intelligent person on earth, but that doesn't make it true. That misses the whole point of what healthy self-talk is all about, though. It's not about where you're at in a particular moment in time, it's about where you want to get to.

If your self-talk isn't helping you then it needs addressing. Simple as. Check whether the words you use to speak to yourself limit you in encouragement, love, helpfulness and progress. I have absolutely no doubt that with consistently healthy and positive self-talk you will achieve more in your life than you would without it – and that is when the evidence comes in! As you achieve more through not limiting yourself with your self-talk, you will see the progress that you are making, which will encourage even more positive self-talk. Suddenly, your words will be backed up by evidence, and the compounding effect of it all will be fucking brilliant!

Sorry . . . here comes that thing again – personal responsibility. I know I am banging on about it, but it is *so* important and it applies to your self-talk massively. You are in charge of how you speak to yourself. It could be empathetic and loving or insulting and harmful, but it is you doing it, no one else. It is also you who can change it. No one is going to supervise you with that or be able to hear what you are saying, because it's all in your head! So, how you do this and how you progress with this is down to you 100 per cent.

Once you become aware of your self-talk, you will also be able to hear it in other people when they speak out loud. You will hear them being down on themselves about something they have done or could achieve. Or maybe they are always moaning about how tired or fed up they are. This may happen with a friend or someone in your family, and you will be able to see how negative they are. It will then become a challenge for you to question whether you want to be near that sort of person regularly. Positive self-talk will drive your mindset, your mindset will drive your behaviours, and your behaviours will drive your outcomes! I am genuinely excited for you if this is something brand new to you and you are going to try it, having read this book. The change for you can be immense!

There is a really important bit of context that I need to add into the topic of self-talk around managing our mental health. The first major bout of depression I suffered from was after my neck operation that eventually forced my retirement. The truth is that up to this point in my life, I didn't really believe in depression. I feel ashamed to say that, but I was naive and had never really experienced it. I had also been living in an environment of extreme positive self-talk, as I have described above, *and* it had worked. I thought depression was a choice, which is terrible to write here, but it's important to be honest. I thought that someone could self-talk themselves out of depression. But then I was hit with it. It was dark and crippling, and I felt totally lost. I couldn't shift it. And this wasn't just some days, it was every day. Looking back, I'm sure there were days prior to that when my mental health wasn't at its best, but nothing like this. A dark cloud just sat on top of me and suffocated me. It was terrible. Truly believing that I should be able to positively self-talk my way out of it – a belief conditioned in my core as an elite athlete – actually made this so much worse because suddenly I couldn't. It was absolutely crushing. Everything that I had trusted with regards to mindset didn't feel real anymore. What was it I said earlier? My mindset would drive my behaviours and my behaviours would drive my outcomes. Well, suddenly my outcomes were fucking shit and there was no way I could get my mindset to a place that would help that out. I had no clue what to do. No clue. It felt like the foundations of my belief system were crumbling.

And that's the thing. The important caveat to all this. There are times when your poor mental health, whether in the form of depression or something else, can be so crippling that self-talk isn't going to work for you at that moment in time; you are going to need more. The way I felt at that time in my life was like nothing I had experienced before, and I don't want anyone reading this chapter who has suffered like that to think that I don't appreciate that. I really do. I also understand that you can practise positive self-talk regularly and still be floored by your mental health at any point in time.

My whole belief system was shaken to the core with regards to the importance of self-talk, and it made me rethink it all. I questioned whether it worked at all, or whether it was a myth that I'd managed to convince myself of in my head. That was really tough because it was something that I'd held onto so tightly all the way to an Olympic medal. I asked myself if all the mindset stuff was nonsense because it hadn't helped me when my mind most needed it. I questioned whether my performances inside the gymnastics arena were mainly down to training and skill – maybe I was just really good at it? If mindset was so important for me then why couldn't it help me when my mind most needed it?

What I came to realise as I started to understand my own mental health challenges was that healthy self-talk is crucial for all human beings. It improves our lives enormously because it is a representation of the love we show ourselves. It frees us from the limitations that our mind can create. My pa, Neil, always says we don't perform to our potential, we perform to the belief of our potential, and it is so true. Negative self-talk narrows our world. It creates fear for us around so much in life. It puts chains around us. It's debilitating. So, it doesn't matter if you are an Olympic athlete or not, how you speak to yourself is massive in helping your life. BUT we mustn't ever expect self-talk to be a cure for mental health issues, as I probably did. That's putting it in a place that misunderstands self-talk and mental health issues in equal measure.

Like everything in this book, positive self-talk is a tool to help you manage your mental health. The more we do it, the more chance we have of keeping away the black clouds of depression and anxiety. I see practising each tool within this book, including healthy self-talk, as a way of creating armour or protection around myself, and I can never get enough of that. My experience of practising this consistently has shown me that my 'dark' days are far fewer than they used to me.

Now I have this clarity in my life, the words 'I can do this' feel even more special to me. They used to be centred around my gymnastics, connected particularly to that Olympic final. I will forever have that beautiful memory, but these words mean even more to me now. They are now an affirmation that 'I can do life', which includes my darkest days with my mental health. I love and care for myself in a way that means I can speak to myself and remind myself that I can do this, I can do life. And I now have evidence to back it up because I have walked through the fire and come out the other side. I can do this and you can do this. Let's just make sure we tell ourselves that a lot!

As I have been writing this book, I have felt a sense of community. I think that's probably because I feel like I am sharing my thoughts with a group of people who understand. It has also reminded me how important community is to human beings. I'm going to talk about this much more in the next chapter and why it's another important factor in our journey of managing our mental health.

WE'RE IN THIS TOGETHER

Humans love humans and, as a result, community is vital to our overall wellbeing.

It can come in different forms and it gives us a sense of belonging and purpose, as well as playing a crucial factor in our growth as individuals. Though it is something that we can take for granted or fail to notice what sort of impact it is having on us. In this chapter, we're going to look at what community actually is, why we are so sensitive to it and how it can play a huge role in helping us to maintain good mental health.

Our most immediate community is our friends and family. We can't choose our family, but I am blessed to have an amazingly loving and supportive one. Though I know this isn't the same for everyone, and that can present lots of complex challenges. It's unlikely to be a straightforward dynamic where difficult relationships with family members are concerned, so all I can say is try to recognise and avoid toxicity in those relationships too if you possibly can. It's worth taking what I tell you in this chapter and seeing if you can adapt that to your family relationships too.

Our friends are a reflection of who we are and where we are at in the world at any given time. I have had a consistent little group of best mates in Luke, Ash and Joey for a long time, and I do think they reflect me. Luke and Ash have been gymnasts, but, more importantly, all three of them are fun and love to laugh. We've had so many mad experiences together, whether filming content, enjoying ourselves in pubs and clubs, or travelling together. They all love to live life to the max and that is very much who I am. I love them all like brothers. I could trust them with anything I tell them and they have always been there for me when I have needed them.

However, that's not to say that there haven't been other people I've socialised with who have not always been the most positive influence on me. Those people were definitely a reflection of where I was at during that time of my life. When I have been in self-destruct mode, I have subconsciously looked for people who can help me with that. Likewise, during that period, I would avoid friends who were trying to warn me away from self-destructive behaviour.

The company that we keep is as much about our needs

and where we are at as anything else. I think that we are all sensitive to our environments, but I don't buy into the phrase 'they are such bad influence on me' – that's just passing the buck. That's the sort of shit I used to say when I was trying to avoid taking responsibility for my actions. When I was at my worst with alcohol and gambling, my two best mates, Luke and Ash, unfairly took some blame for it. People thought it was their influence on me, but that wasn't true. It was me versus me and they were often trying to look after me without being able to control me. Everything I did came down to decisions that I was making – no one else. So, sorry guys, it's that personal responsibility thing again – we can just never get away from it!

The healthiest friendship groups have balance and respect. There has to be an equilibrium that makes you feel safe to express who you are. Ash is a former British gymnast and was a teammate of mine at Leeds Gymnastics Club. We have literally spent hours upon hours with each other training, travelling and competing. Ash was a far more talented gymnast than me but I was fortunate enough to do better in competitions. Ash suffered with some bad injuries and I think I just excelled when I was performing. But having said that, there has never been a 'better' or 'worse' within our friendship; we were just two lads from Leeds experiencing so much together. Our lives have been intertwined by gymnastics but our friendship has never been about comparison, just love and support. We pushed each other in training and inspired each other at different times, but the foundation of it all has just been a deep unconditional friendship, nothing else. I have been able to share with Ash exactly where I'm at and not worry about judgement or looking stupid.

A big part of looking after our mental health is having close friends that we can feel safe enough to share this with. Friends who will love and support you if you are struggling, rather than judge. Friends who will understand if you need to stay off the booze or stay away from certain places for a period of time. If there is any level of toxicity in these friend-ships then they can't be right for you. The easiest way to judge whether this is the case is to ask yourself whether those friends make you truly happy and healthy in life. If they don't then there is toxicity there to avoid.

Surround yourself with people who lift you up and don't pull you down with cynicism or destructiveness. Look for people who will be as caring with you when you're on the way down as they were when you were on your way up in life. Who want to hang out when you are not at your best as well as when you are on great form. True friendship is recip-rocal, where you help each other's needs, and if it isn't then you really have to ask yourself what you are doing.

I see far too many people being caught in one-way, unhealthy or toxic friendships because they con themselves that it is about loyalty and longstanding relationships, but the truth is that doesn't make any sense. Why would you continue a relationship that diminishes you as a person? You are making a choice to do something that undermines your own sense of worth and esteem. You might have known each other forever or feel like you have shared a lot in the past, but if a relationship is unhealthy, all it will do is limit how good you can be as a person, which is going to harm who you'll be for the loved ones in your life. They deserve the best version of you.

Take a moment now to think about your friendship group in the present and past.

- Does it have or has it had that safety and equilibrium that I've talked about above?
- Who has been there when you have been super happy and who has been there when you were going through a more troubled time?
- When you meet up with one or some of your friends, what information do you share? Is it full of fear and dread or is it full of light and optimism?

As you do think about these things, remember that this investigation is about *you*, not them.

We are all influenced by the environments in which we find ourselves (or, more accurately, place ourselves), and I always remind myself of the quote 'if you go to the barbers enough then eventually you'll get a haircut'. In other words, the more you are in a certain environment, the more you will morph into that. All of the conversations we have and the information we listen to, watch or read impact our mental health. Our closest friends are an important part of this. The more information I consume that fills me with fear, the more terrified I am of what is around the corner in life. That does nothing for my mental health. For example, you might have friendships where there is no doubt that your friend cares for you, but the way they view and talk about the world really pulls you down. It is a reciprocal relationship, but ultimately not that healthy for you. You have to seriously consider whether that is a friendship you need to spend a lot of time in or find some distance from.

It is also important to broaden your horizons in terms of the people you speak to and engage with, so that you can learn from others who have seen more of the world or are more knowledgeable in certain areas. It's good to be challenged in that way and I've always been super inspired to meet people who can tell me things that I have never heard about before. I just want to absorb every bit of information I can from them.

I love talking about business with the other shareholders at Nile Wilson Gymnastics, which is our business opening gymnastics clubs around the world. Likewise, I love talking to other athletes and content creators, like Ross Edgeley.

Ross and I have been friends for a long time and filmed a fitness challenge video on YouTube back in 2017 that went viral. Since then, Ross has done some truly incredible things, including swimming all the way around Great Britain in 2018, which blows my fucking mind! He swam for 157 days in some brutal conditions, and what that man knows about endurance, determination and self-will is something that we all need in our lives. Ross is definitely someone I want to talk to as much as possible. Every conversation I have with him inspires me and I learn so much. His knowledge of the human body and what it is capable of is incredible, and he has this energy about life that makes me want to get out there and achieve things. But here's the thing – Ross isn't in my inner circle of friends, and so the point I'm trying to make is that this is not just about your inner circle; your wider community is super important too. I sometimes think the two things get muddled up, and in recent times, I have really started to understand why all of us need community in our lives, particularly when it comes to managing our mental health. Much of what I have seen in this area always focuses on that inner circle, but I think it's bigger than that.

Community, in my eyes, is being part of a group of people who give you friendship, influence, support, knowledge, purpose and, most importantly, a sense of belonging. This group can come from where you live or what you do, like a sport, a club, a church, a project, a business, a charity – basically anything that brings people together to go after and achieve common goals. Ross is part of my content creator, elite athlete, mad challenger community!

Humans need community in their lives, and if ever you need proof of that then we just need to look at the gigantic mental health issues that stemmed from lockdown during Covid. When human beings are isolated from their communities, we find life very difficult. Humans need humans. I see around me all the time how we come together in tribes. Just look at football and supporting a particular club – that's all about having a tribe or community to belong to. Even the mad world of politics is all about people wanting to feel attached to a cause and be part of a group of people who feel the same way as they do. Basically, I just think we all find the world really overwhelming at times and community helps us to feel more secure and stable.

What are the community or communities around you? Do they help you grow as a person in one way or another? The fact that you are reading this book will certainly mean you are interested in being part of a community of people who are trying to understand their mental health better.

I'm going to give you two examples of community in my life, which are very different in nature. The first is me joining my local golf club, Headingley Golf Club. I love golf. I am completely addicted to the challenge of it. But arguably I could play golf on my own, so what does being a member of the club give me? Well, I become part of a golfing community where I get to meet new people, play in competitions, chat with other members in the clubhouse over food and drinks, have more time with my dad and learn how to play the sport better. My dad has been a member of the club for 37 years (can you believe that?!), and there's now a group of about 20 of us who play every week, go on golf trips together and have become really good friends. It gives me everything that I believe community is all about.

My second example is *very* different. Alcoholics Anonymous is a community of people who are trying to help each other overcome their addiction to alcohol. The entire premise of the organisation is that people with greater experience help those who have newly arrived. For someone in their early days of recovery, this is priceless. They feel less alone in their battle with addiction and receive the benefit of guidance from people who have trodden the path before them. Likewise, for the 'older' members helping the 'younger' ones, this gives them purpose and direction with something they feel enormously passionate about. By helping people who are in much earlier days of sobriety, they are reminded of the important principles that they learned to get and stay healthy. It is a true community where everyone is helping each other to grow in life. It's a very different example to me being a member of my golf club, but the same dynamics of community apply.

Sports clubs are obvious examples of communities, but so are book clubs, dance groups, wine clubs, drama clubs or any sort of therapy/support group someone might be part of. What do you have around you right now that represents a community? If you're struggling for an answer here then it's something that I would really like you to look at. The benefits that come from joining the right sort of community will be huge for you. I would actually be incredibly excited for you to take that step.

In the same way that I said our close circle of friends is a reflection on where we are at as human beings at any given moment, so is whether we are truly engaged in a community or not. It can feel daunting to go and join a club or group, but it is a massive statement to make to yourself, as much as anyone. It might take time to actively engage with other people within that club or group, but that's OK; it would be a step to try to broaden your horizons. It is also another way to show the personal responsibility you are taking for improving your situation in life. You're not waiting for someone or something to come to you; you're getting yourself out there to be part of a community that could really help you. I genuinely don't think there is any downside in this for you.

As I come to the end of this chapter, I want to share with you what my head tells me when I am really struggling with my mental health. It tells me to hide in a corner from the rest of the world, curl up in a little ball and cry. It tells me that the world is to be feared and I can't cope with it. It tells me that I am a failure and a weak person. It tells me that there is nothing worth living for. It tells me that I am far better off on my own than with anyone else. It strips away every bit of connection I have in my life, and the more I listen to it, the worse it gets. Humans need humans – we need connection. A healthy group of close friends is crucial for this but so is an extended community or communities to feel part of. They represent the exact antidote to the darkness and loneliness that poor mental health can give us. So, if you haven't already, then get out there and find your tribes or your communities in life!

This entire chapter has very much focused on what we get or receive from our friends or community, but there is something crucial missing from this. One of the most important lessons I have learned in recent times is that what I/we offer to our friends or communities is absolutely vital to our mental health. It's not so much about what we receive and more about what we give to it. That is what we are going to delve into in the next chapter.

LESS ME AND MORE WE

Altruism. I'm honest enough to tell you that two years ago I had no idea what this word meant. Now, when I say this, there's two parts to this. I literally didn't know what it meant, as in looking in a dictionary type stuff, but, maybe more importantly, I didn't come close to understanding the true meaning of it up until about 12 months ago.

For those of you who don't know, here's the definition of altruism via the Oxford Dictionary: 'the fact of caring about the needs and happiness of other people and being willing to do things to help them, even if it brings no advantage to yourself.'

Seems easy enough, right? It's basically doing something for someone else without getting anything back. We do it all the time! We buy presents, open doors, give people lifts to places, let people in front of us, etc, etc. I've always felt like

I've been a pretty decent person and done all these sorts of things, so I guessed that I'd been practising altruism. But then that final part of the definition was pointed out to me – 'even if it brings no advantage to yourself'. Well, I would think to myself that when I open a door for someone, I'm not looking for anything back, am I? But . . . is that really true?

How many of us get annoyed when someone doesn't say thank you when we have opened a door for them? I certainly have. In which case, then, I was looking for something back for my good deed. It might not have been a physical act in return, but in a situation like this, in my mind, I had made an invisible transaction with someone: 'I open the door and you say thank you for my good deed.' That's not altruism. This is something I talked about in the chapter 'Why Not Me', when we looked at the concept of 'self-serving'. Our focus can be subconsciously on ourselves even when we are doing acts for other people. We think we're being selfless but our intentions are not that pure. Understanding and practising altruism has played a huge role in helping my mental health, and it can do the same for you too.

How many of our kind acts in life contain an invisible transaction like the one above that we don't even acknowledge to ourselves? Do we do kind things for people because we actually want recognition from them, either in terms of receiving a return act for ourselves ('you owe me') or affirmation that we are good people? If you're anything like me then you'll be shocked how often you answer 'yes' to this question.

I remember the first time I was confronted by this and suddenly thought about the phrase 'unconditional love'. It's a term that's thrown around a lot, but how often is it actually practised? Unconditional means without conditions, without any transaction. But without ever consciously thinking about it, I had been making silent deals throughout my life. Even the words 'I love you' – how often do we say them because we want the other person to say them back to us? I definitely have. It's the most sacred and beautiful thing to say to someone else and, in actual fact, we sometimes say it because we just want something back! That's mad. I can think of loads of times that I have bought a big, extravagant present for someone because, if I'm truly honest, I have wanted it to be a reflection of me – i.e. that I have money and/or that I am a really good and generous person. It's mind-blowing when you really think about it. I shock myself with how much selfishness can sit within me even when I am doing 'kind' things. The more you really analyse this in yourself, the more you'll be able to see it everywhere.

How often do you ask a friend how they are because you are secretly using it as an intro for them to ask you how you are?

How often do you put something on social media that

appears kind, but you actually crave the attention you'll get back for doing so?

How often do you appear to be kind but there is actually something in it for you?

These are really uncomfortable questions to ask yourself, but do it! No one is listening or needs to know your answers so you can be brutally honest with yourself. I know it might make you feel bad initially, but I promise it's worth it.

I guess you might now ask what this has to do with managing our mental health, and even why does it make a difference in any case? Surely kindness is just kindness and always a good thing? Well, you are sort of right. Kindness *is* always a good thing, but this discussion is not about the actual kind act or gesture, it is about what is going through our heads throughout all of this.

The easiest way I can describe this is by talking about my own experience. I was asked once whether I saw the world as something that I should be taking from or something that I should be giving to – was I a consumer or a contributor? That was a tough question for a lad in this early twenties from Leeds who wanted to conquer the world! Of course I wanted to grab things! The world just looked like a landscape of opportunity for me then and there was so much for me to achieve. And do you know what? I still feel like that. But there is something subtle within this that I never appreciated. The question about how I saw the world was based on where my primary focus was. Was it to 'take' or to 'give'? If it was all on what I could get from the world then it was always going to be about what was in it for me. I'm not saying this was a conscious thing, but, nonetheless, it was there in my mind and so of course had a big impact on my acts of 'kindness'.

So, what was so wrong with this? Well, poor mental health wants you stuck in your own dark thoughts. It wants to isolate you. It wants you to look no further than the confines of what you believe you need and want in life. It wants you to stay completely self-absorbed. If we live in a mindset that the world is 'all about me', whether consciously or subconsciously, then we are much more likely to fall into poor mental health than if we look more to what we could 'give' to the world and others around us.

In essence, we are already isolating ourselves due to our selfishness, because our view is that life is always measured by what we get. And, in that case, there are going to be constant ups and downs because it is impossible to always get what we want or think we deserve. If that's our metric for how life is going then we are in trouble.

I could never see or understand this until it was explained to me in these terms. We can still, and in fact I would encourage you to, view the world as full of opportunity for things we can enjoy and achieve. There is nothing wrong with that but, alongside it, we need an appreciation that it can't be all one-way traffic. It can't all be about us being the consumer. This line has always stuck to sum this up:

Be of service because you want to be enthralled by the world, not because you want the world to be enthralled by you.

In other words, do good things because it will make you appreciate and connect you with the world so much more than if you are just performing good deeds because you want everyone to think how great you are.

In my opinion, a wider appreciation for what we are offering to the world, rather than hoping to take from it, is absolutely vital for maintaining good mental health. The reason for this is because we start to measure the quality of our life through a different lens. We're not judging success just on the ups and downs of whether we get what we want at any given time – instead we are measuring our lives based on the purity of our intentions to help others without anything in return. If we are doing that and being the best person that we can be, then there can be no other expectation that we can place on ourselves.

We can still go out there and try to achieve everything we want to in life. We can still want to grab every opportunity we can, but it is not our only measurable. If it is then there will never be an 'enough'. When we buy ourselves that new car, new phone, new clothes or new whatever it is – that's just a material achievement that makes us feel good for a fleeting moment. The same goes with the next medal, the next business deal, the next zero in a bank balance, the next view on social media – it will never be enough and at a certain point we will need that next high. But when we can serve and think of other people, we can start to see the good that comes to us beyond our own needs. I know that to find true fulfilment in my life I have to make it about more than just myself.

There is also a practical angle to all of this when you're struggling with your mental health. Like I said earlier, poor mental health wants to isolate you, and I have learned that a simple trick to get out of my own head is to ask someone else how they are. For example, if I start to feel myself getting low and wanting to hide away, and then I reach out to someone else and ask them how their day is going, my mind immediately starts to focus on them rather than myself. I sort of un-isolate myself! I don't have to tell them about how I am feeling, but it often comes up eventually. The most important point is that I find a way of not getting lost in my own thoughts and instead switch my focus to someone else. If you're not used to this then it will take some practice, but it is well worth it.

So, the important question is, how are you 'being of service' in your life?

I'm sure that has just prompted a 'what the fucking hell does that mean?!' Ha-ha, yeah, I get it – 'being of service' does sound a bit weird, but just bear with me! 'Being of service' basically means exactly what we have just been talking about – doing things for other people in our lives without any benefit returning to us. In other words: altruism.

Ask yourself now if there are areas in your life in which you are truly doing this. If you are anything like I was then the cupboard might be a little bare to start with on this front! I think you might find this to be much tougher than you first assume. For example, how many of you hoover your house and then tell your partner that you've done it because you want some recognition for it? How many of you find a mistake made by a work colleague, correct it and then tell them you've done so because you want them to know that you've fixed their mess? How many of you do a favour for a friend thinking that one day they'll need to repay that debt to you? Honestly, there are so many examples.

The 30-day altruism challenge

I'm going to set you a challenge so you can test yourself with this. The test starts today and runs for 30 days. I want you to do a good thing for someone else in the world every day of this challenge and never tell them. I don't mean something good for the same person for 30 days, but a kind act every day for someone and keep it a secret. Now, when I say never tell them, I really mean *never*! You can't tell them at the time, or after the 30 days, or at any point ever in the future. Every day is to be a kind secret that you keep to yourself. When you embark on this you are going to see how hard it is not to self-seek for recognition. If it's not something you are used to, like I wasn't, then it is a fucking shock to the system, but it is a brilliant way of learning how to be of service to others in a truly altruistic way.

'Being of service' in your life actually starts with those closest to you, and I have had to really get honest about this with myself. My family are so supportive of me and always have been. My parents and my sister gave me unconditional love and support throughout my entire gymnastics career and often sacrificed their needs for mine. My sister spent a good chunk of her childhood hanging out at gymnastics clubs because I was there doing the sport, *not* her. And they still very much continue to do this for me today with my business ventures and my YouTube channel. But the question is how often has my first thought been about what they need rather than what I need? Well, the truth is that it has too often been about what I want rather than what they need. I have had to catch myself on this so often and, in many ways, relearn my thinking around it.

The irony of it all is that this basically goes against everything that you develop as an elite athlete, when it is all about you. It used to be all about my training and competitions and what I needed – I was so focused on gymnastics that everything else came in a distant second place, whether it was family, girlfriend or anything else. But I have discovered that way of living isn't sustainable if you want to enjoy a healthy life. If there is a major goal that requires all your energy – like the Olympics for me – then there might be times when your mind is all on one thing. But that can't last forever, and what you are left with at the end of it is not a healthy mental state.

I have learned that life can be as simple or as complicated as we want to make it. If I wake up every day with a list of things that I want and expect from the world then it all becomes very complicated. With constant expectations come lots of disappointments because nothing in life is simple or, more importantly, ever enough. Our mental health will seriously suffer in that headspace. Whereas if I wake up with the sole focus of being the best human being I can be then life is beautifully simple. That doesn't mean I am some sort of doormat with no real ambition in the world, absolutely not, but my focus is different. Being the best version of myself also includes being smart and hardworking; it's just that underneath that lies a foundation of what I am all about that keeps me healthy. I can take a moment at the start of each day to think about how I can be of service to others. My family and friends are obvious starting points, but just as important is how I am when I walk into a café full of people, for example. Am I being attentive to anyone who needs help or giving the person serving a respectful amount of attention, or am I simply staring at my phone while lost in my own head? That's a choice I can make, that we can all make, to stay mentally healthy.

This isn't about becoming a martyr to others, by the way! I'm not asking you to sacrifice all your needs for the sake of other people. I am asking you to look at how you measure your life through your intentions. Being of service to other people can't be at the detriment to your own health. If you're not healthy then you can't help others – it's as simple as that. You need to consider whether the service you are giving fits with your lifestyle, your ability and your time and energy capacity. There is no point embarking on something that will end up being self-defeating.

Likewise, you have to consider why it's important to you. Being of service isn't about box ticking. If you want to help that person in the café who is struggling to get a buggy out of the door then do it because it's important to you to help others. Also, have a think about whether the help you want to give someone else is at the right moment in time. They might not want to receive it when you want to give it! You might want to cheer up a friend who is having a bad week but maybe they aren't ready yet. Sometimes a big part of being of service to someone else is waiting for them to be ready to receive help, rather than you deciding it is their time to get it.

The last point to consider is to not overcomplicate your life – keep things simple. I have talked about how we can make life complicated or simple with our intentions; well, don't create huge difficulties for yourself by trying to be of service. In my experience, helping others should be quite simple because it's more often than not about the small acts on the quiet when no one notices. If you find that everything is becoming overly complicated then it might not be the right thing to do. Again, ask yourself if you're trying to do something that isn't going to be healthy for you.

I want to finish by giving you this quote from Mahatma Gandhi: 'The best way to find yourself is to lose yourself in the service of others.' Take some time now to think about your life and how often you are of complete service to others. How does it make you feel when you do it? Can you do it more? Maybe you're not doing it at all?

I hope I have given you some food for thought on how to realign your focus and intentions in life. I am going to continue this into the next chapter and challenge you to rethink your definition of success. This might sound strange coming from an ex-Olympian but hear me out!

WIN OR LOSE, RIGHT?

Defining success should be fairly simple, right?

You get the job or you don't get the job.

You finish the race or you don't finish the race.

You close out the business deal or you don't close out the business deal.

You get the medal or you don't get the medal.

You win or you lose, simple.

As an elite athlete, I have grown up in a world where that is very much the definition of success and I have built so many of my life experiences around this. Success is a binary thing within elite performance – you either achieve the thing you set out to achieve or you fail to. And it's not just a theory or opinion, it's an attitude built around not making excuses and shooting for the very best every single time you perform. There is a hardness to it that drives you forward when things get tough. By making sure there is no middle

163

ground, you get rid of any softness or mediocrity. It's the life professional sportspeople operate in and it's very effective. We push ourselves to extreme levels and, as a consequence, extraordinary results are achieved. Performances are produced that shock and inspire people. Athletes overcome torturous setbacks through the most mind-blowing mental toughness because they will not accept, under any circumstances, that they will not be successful in that moment. The flip side of it, of course, is that we also see the extreme heartbreak when an athlete doesn't achieve success. Their pain comes out of every part of their being because they have put *everything* on the line to win. There are no half measures. It's harsh, it's brutal, but it is what elite performance is built on and, as spectators, we love it.

Maybe not for the first time in this book, I might be about to shock you. I want us to rethink everything I have told you above. In short, I want us to redefine how we measure success in life. The reason for this is that one of the most important lessons I've learned in recent years is that this attitude to success can seriously fuck with your mental health. I fully appreciate that I am saying something that goes completely against the grain of the sporting environment in which I achieved so much success, and so, before we tackle this redefining of success, I will need to explain to you why I am asking you to do this.

In many ways, the example of elite sport and, more

specifically, the Olympics is a perfect illustration of the point I want to make on this.

My journey to one day making history at the 2016 Rio Olympics for British Gymnastics probably started when I was about seven years old. About three years after I first started gymnastics, people around me – specifically my parents and my coaches – began to realise that I was really good at it. Even at that age, it was clear that I was very talented, incredibly competitive and had the courage to try anything. I think I probably started to realise all that around the same time as well. I knew I was far better than almost every other kid doing the sport alongside me.

Back then, my first club, Leeds Gymnastics Club, was based at the Carnegie University in Headingley and was run by a man called Mike Talbot or, as we used to call him, 'Mr T'! Mr T was an amazing man and I was so lucky to have him involved in my early gymnastics. He had a genuine love for the sport and his passion was infectious. I loved all my sessions with him. Mr T fast-tracked me into being a full member of the club. Back then, to get into Leeds Gymnastics Club, you would ordinarily need to impress in a regional competition, but Mr T just ignored that. In fact, one day, he pointed at me in front of all the other kids and said, 'That kid's special. Really special.' I was identified early on as a potential gymnastics star, which happens a lot in sports like gymnastics where you need to bloom early. There are no such things as 'late starters' in gymnastics.

So, whether we knew it or not, my family and I began an Olympic dream journey from that point in time. Everything began to be geared around me and what I needed for my gymnastics. My ma was forever taxiing me back and forth to training and my sister would do her homework at the gymnastics club while I trained. The expectation level around me was always super high because we could all see what I was capable of. I think that subconsciously we were all aiming for me to reach the peak of Everest – the Olympic Games. For a gymnast, there is nothing higher than the Olympics – it really is what dreams are made of.

As my junior gymnastics gathered momentum and I made it into the national squads as well as doing well in major competitions, the Olympic dream started to crystalise. It's incredible how much of your life gets laser focused around it. I remember watching all the hype and excitement around the London 2012 Olympics when I was sixteen years old and genuinely thinking that could be me in four years' time. There is no question that it is an incredibly special target, and if you realise it then it is life-changing. But the thing no one notices at the time is that it is a target with specific end points.

You either make the Olympic team or you don't.

The Games will last for a set period of time.

You will either win a medal or you won't.

People rarely consider what comes after it. Yeah, sure, you could argue that what comes after it is another Olympic Games, but that's not right around the corner. It is another four-year cycle of absolute dedication and then you *might* make the team if your form is still excellent and you're not injured. Also, eventually, there won't be another Olympics in you. So, the question of what is next if you do reach the peak of Everest in a sporting context is something people don't talk about often enough while you're climbing up it.

What does actually come next for Olympians is a massive crash. I don't know an Olympian who hasn't come home from the Games and not experienced some sort of massive mental comedown. The incredible swimmer Adam Peaty calls it the 'Olympic blues'.

I will never forget returning to Leeds after the Rio Olympics. I had a history-making bronze medal and felt on top of the world. I partied non-stop in Rio as soon as my competing was over and I felt like I was on cloud nine. I had been fulfilling loads of media commitments and my phone was just non-stop with congratulatory messages from people. I was still living with my parents at the time, and after a couple of nights at home, I woke up late and came downstairs to find that my ma had quite reasonably left me a to-do list of jobs around the house. Fuck, it hit me hard – I was an Olympic medallist, a huge dream had come true for me, and yet here I was, standing in the kitchen, looking at a list that included when I needed to hang up the washing. Talk about coming crashing back down to earth!

But it wasn't just that. The Olympics is like the biggest explosion of emotions in which you experience massive dopamine highs. But then suddenly you land back in the normality of everyday life. You have worked all your life to achieve your dream and then you are back to to-do lists, arguments with your girlfriend and getting frustrated with the traffic. There's nothing wrong with that as such, but you are just not prepared for the crash back to reality. People don't really talk about that when aiming for the peak of the mountain – and why would they? The chase is far too exciting.

Whether it is called the 'Olympic blues' or anything else, there is definitely a massive effect on an athlete's mental health. I guess it's understandable with the extreme change in emotions, the sudden loss of purpose and the fact that life is still life. It doesn't even matter if you have won or lost, everyone experiences that crash. Michael Phelps, who is arguably the greatest Olympian of all time with 28 Olympic medals to his name, suffered from severe bouts of depression in between every Olympics he competed in and has admitted, after the London 2012 Olympics, to having strong suicidal thoughts before entering a treatment centre.

I know my example with the Olympics is a rare and

extreme one, but the lessons it taught me around how we define success apply to all areas of my life now, and I believe they apply in the same way for you as well. The reason why the Olympics crash is so strong is that up to the point that it happens, everything, and I mean *everything*, is pointed towards achieving the 'goal'. Like I said earlier, there is a specific end point to it all. And this applies to so much in our lives.

Are you fixated on earning a certain amount of money, of getting a particular job, moving to a specific place, getting a boyfriend or girlfriend, losing or gaining an amount of weight or being able to afford a certain car or other material items? If you are then they all have a specific end point – and you either achieve them or you don't. What often comes after that, whether you got the thing you wanted or not, is what I can best describe as flatness. You're not chasing any-more and perhaps that thing isn't as life-changing as you thought it would be. Maybe you don't know what to do with yourself now.

That is what happens when your goal that you define as 'success' has an end point. The only answer to the flatness is to set a new target, and the cycle continues until it can no longer. Then you experience a sense of nothingness again. What comes after every mini or major chase can have a mas-sively detrimental impact on our mental health. Finally understanding this has been so useful in terms of figuring out how to manage my mental health after retiring from gymnastics. I can see so clearly that the model elite sport gave me isn't workable outside of it and that if I constantly judge my success by an end-point goal and nothing else then I am in trouble.

So, to maintain a level of stability with my mental wellbeing and general happiness, my life needs to be centred around a different definition of success. At the moment, my company is opening gymnastics clubs all around the country and growing fast. It is incredibly exciting and all the people closest to me are involved. We are making amazing progress and aim to have ten to fifteen clubs open within the next five years. Each club has around a thousand children taking part in gymnastics and I am so proud of it. Yes, there is a clear opportunity for me to do well financially out of this business, but if I want to stay happy and healthy and help keep this project thriving then I have to keep enjoying it. My focus can't be on an end point or a financial milestone for all the reasons that I have stated above.

I've realised that while elite sport may have ingrained in me a binary definition of succeed/fail, I still loved learning and then mastering a new gymnastics skill. The joy was in getting better; I wasn't constantly thinking about what score it would get in a competition. The key is that I have to be in love with the process rather than the end result. When I am focused on making kids smile in the gym, listening to parents, helping to develop the coaches and generally being of service to everyone involved, then I am getting so much out of it without a benchmark achievement in sight. Seeing new kids arrive, learn and have an incredible time, while the coaches are blossoming as people while they teach them – it's completely amazing. I don't focus on the amount of money going into the bank account and create targets around that.

So, how do I redefine success within this context? Well, I don't see it as an end point. Success comes from whether I am being the best I can be within the process. I ask myself whether I have been of service to everyone at Nile Wilson Gymnastics, and if the answer is yes then I am winning. It doesn't mean I have *won*; it means that I am winning. The important lessons I learned about altruism – whether we view the world as something we take from or give to – that I talked about in the previous chapter have massively fed into this. I now know that if I judge my success by my intentions then I feel unshakable because it is all centred on a process rather than an end result. There will be some things that go very well in my life and some that won't, but I'm OK with that as long as I know my intentions were where they should have been and I worked at enjoying the process. These days, that is my definition of 'winning'.

OK, so now let's ask how you can start to question your

definition of success and realign it, if necessary, to something that guides you and helps you feel fulfilled in your life. I hope that during this chapter, you have already had a few lightbulb moments about how you approach success in your life, but there are two areas in particular that I would like you to have a close look at.

Your work

Is your approach to your job dominated by a particular promotion you want or a particular salary/bonus you hope to achieve? Or are you in love with and absorbed by the actual work involved? If your answer is yes to the latter and no to the former, then you're in the right place. You will blossom within that environment because you appreciate the processes that are involved in your work. If your answer was no to the latter and yes to the former, then you do seriously need to think about finding different work. In these instances, someone can say to me, 'Well, that's easy for you to say but I need the money.' I understand that and I know that is often someone's reality, but then just acknowledge the compromise you are making and that it's really not good if this remains the case in the long term. If your work is all about the end result of the money you get then it is going to eat away at your mental health. Whether we like it or not, we spend a lot of our lives working, and it is a key place for us to manage our mental health is a positive way.

Money

This is actually a pretty deep set of questions to ask yourself, but do you see money as bringing you status in life? Do you see it as a marker of how successful you are? Does it dominate your thinking with regards to what direction to take in life? Money is important in all our lives, there's no getting away from that. Little money means few options and lots of money often means the luxury of choice. But our relationship with money says so much about our definition of success and how we view life in general. Money provides us with endless end-point goals – e.g. I'll retire when I make that amount of money; or, when I earn that salary, everything will be sorted in my life; or, when I can afford to buy that, I'll be happy; or, because I have this amount of money, people should respect me.

I've fallen into these traps myself and learned some of my hardest life lessons with money. I have been fortunate and smart enough to generate some significant amounts of money in my life, but every time I have focused on a monetary end point, life has given me a sharp lesson around it.

I once dreamed about owning a penthouse apartment in Leeds and now I do. I saw it as a place that would signify the money I had made and how successful I was, and yet, though I was finally able to buy that apartment, it was the place in which my gambling, drinking and mental health were at their worst.

I used to fantasise about having an incredible car and I eventually bought one. I thought I would look so cool in it and it would be another reflection of my money and success. It was in that car that I got a 12-month driving ban and had to pay out a ton of money in fines and legal costs. These were two big things in my life that I knew would be achieved by a certain amount of money and I was sure would result in a certain amount of happiness and status for me. The reality was the opposite.

I love being successful in life and I'm as motivated as I have ever been, but how I define success has changed immensely in the last two years. I have learned this through pain and poor decisions (which I would rather you avoided!), and I have begun to understand that there is a place in life where I can be consistently happy while trying to achieve great things, rather than placing myself on a rollercoaster of metrics of what I believe 'success' *should* look like. I absorb myself in the journey and the process of trying to achieve certain things and, as a result, I love it all, wherever it takes me.

Take time to reflect on your perception of what success looks like and whether what I have said in this chapter has resonated with you.

Are you constantly chasing things in the belief that the next win will make everything better?

Having achieved successes, have you ever found the feeling of satisfaction to be short lived?

Challenge yourself on this and see if it is something that needs some realignment in your life.

We have talked about emotions a lot throughout this book, and it's because I want you to become self-aware of how you feel in given moments and how that can affect you mentally. That awareness gives you an understanding of how you want to react from that emotion. In this next chapter, I am going to talk you through one very powerful emotion and how we can use it to benefit our mental health.

WHEN YOU'RE AFRAID, GOOD SHIT HAPPENS

Feeling afraid is one of the most primitive emotions we have.

There's good reason for this in some ways – from the sabre-toothed tiger chasing the caveman to crossing the road when a fast car is approaching, feeling fear is an important warning sign for human beings. But, importantly, fear needs careful management in our lives. When we experience high levels of anxiety, fear can cripple. But there is a way to manage fear that can drive us forward rather than diminish us. In this chapter, I am going to show you how and encourage you to embrace this.

As human beings, we need movement. We need literal movement to stay healthy, but we also need movement in terms of how we grow in our lives through experiences, knowledge and relationships. It's part of being a healthy person. Without it, we can get stuck, lost and isolated – and even feel like we are going backwards. But here's the thing: to be able to keep moving forward in your life, you are going to feel afraid at times. You are going to have to feel uncomfortable and be able to step through it. This is so important for your mental wellbeing. So, rather than this be a warning message from me, I want it to be an encouraging message – I wish for you to be afraid at times in life. It's healthy for all of us.

I have felt a healthy amount of fear millions of times in my life. I felt it every time I stood at the start of a tumble on a floor routine, about to do a 'double double', which is a double twisting, double somersault. I have done it hundreds of times, but I would always feel that fear before I set off because there was a chance that it could go horribly wrong. I could mess it up, and the routine, and the whole competition – but worse, I could land on my fucking head! I experienced the same kind of fear constantly when I was doing *Dancing on Ice*, as I was pushing the limits as to what skills I could perform in a sport that was brand new to me. That fear can be such a powerful driver in making sure you go for it – but you have to embrace it.

I was asked to give a TED Talk in Prague in 2022, which was a real honour and something I had always wanted to do, but I had never done anything like that. Well, not really. I had given speeches in the past, but not on the scale and with the prestige of a TED Talk. This was going to go online and would be there forever, rather than just be something I said at an awards ceremony. Also, TED Talks have to be an exact length and are filmed live, so you can't fuck it up.

I was given about six months to prepare for it, but in true Wilsonator style, actually gave myself about six days to prepare for it! My friends and family came to Prague with me, and 48 hours before the event, I was shitting myself. I was horribly underprepared and I suddenly felt the enormity of what I was about to do, but . . . I STEPPED THROUGH IT. I embraced that feeling and recognised it as something healthy rather than scary. I stayed in my hotel room for 24 hours practising my talk over and over again, using positive self-talk and visualisation, just like I described in the chapter 'Me Versus Me'.

There was another kicker in this talk for me because it was titled 'What Can Make Me an Olympic Champion Can Also Kill Me'. It was going to be a talk that shocked people because I would expose how my personality, talent and nature can give me great strengths in life but can also hurt me. It was very much in line with a lot of what I have written about in this book. I had to get it right and, of course, I felt fear around it, just as I did at the start of a tumble on my floor routine.

As I walked up on stage in Prague, I felt nervous and excited. But I recognised that those feelings were good ones to have. I was about to do something that would help me grow. It was challenging – that's why I felt afraid; I was not under threat. Whatever happened, I knew that I would learn and evolve as a person. It wasn't as intense as stepping up to perform my high bar routine in the Olympic final, but there was a similarity about it. I said to myself, 'I can do this,' and I knew that the whole thing was good for me as a person.

The talk went fantastically well and I loved it. I didn't deliver the speech exactly how I had planned, but no one noticed. I felt really proud about it and I still do today when I watch it back. The thing is that I felt proud in how I delivered it, but I felt even prouder about the fact that it was another experience in life that had frightened me but I had embraced it and moved forward. The reality is that I have been doing this so much in my life that I'm now a bit addicted to it! If there is something that gives me that feeling of being afraid then I want to take it on. Rather than pushing me away, it attracts me to it. Some people might describe me as brave to do some of the things I do, but that's not because I don't experience fear, I just see it positively – and I want you to see it this way too.

How we control or manage our fear is so fundamental to us in understanding how to maintain good mental health. The ability to control our fear comes from us recognising where it comes from. When we are just about to go for that job interview, or perform in some way, or meet someone for the first time and we feel a little afraid, it is because our mind is being dominated by 'WHAT IF'. For example, 'what if I get this wrong?', 'what if they don't like me?' or 'what if I forget my lines?' We don't like not knowing what the result of something will be and we worry that it could go the way we don't want it to, and about what the consequences of that would be. But just imagine if you got to a place mentally where you knew that *whatever* the result, everything would be OK – even great. It's not to say you won't still feel some fear, but that you recognise it comes from you trying something out of your comfort zone.

I want you to start to reframe that feeling of being afraid into something very different. Trying brand new things in life should scare you a little! We all remember trying to ride a bike for the first time and none of us did that without feeling scared – it's perfectly normal. But imagine now that the 'WHAT IF' element of it was the best part of it all. Yes, *what if* the uncertainty was actually the icing on the cake of the experience? In fact, imagine that this was so much the case that the fear you felt was a signal that what you were about to do would be absolutely brilliant for you.

Without getting too philosophical, I want to share with you what Buddha said about uncertainty: all things are inherently transient whether life is stable or totally off-kilter at any point in time. When we really think about this we can understand that uncertainty is part of life. Certainty in life is an illusion – or, more accurately, wanting to be certain about life is a fool's errand. You can never truly know what the outcome is going to be. The goal is to be able to feel comfortable when facing uncertain results. Things do go wrong in life; it's part of life's journey, part of the normal uncertainty of life. If we can take this on board then we can start to see that all new experiences in life are good for us.

Can you look back on things that happened to you in the last few years that seemingly went wrong but ended up being an enormous blessing in disguise? Maybe there was a job you didn't get which meant you ended up getting another one you now love, or forced you to have a much needed change in direction? Maybe there was a relationship break-up which felt horrendous at the time, but now you look back on it and realise that it was right to have ended? Maybe there was a performance that didn't go so well that forced you to address some things you needed to and improved you immeasurably?

If you're anything like me then you will have had loads of experiences like this in life. So, can you remember this when you are about to embark on something new that scares you a little? If you can then you could reach a place mentally that doesn't only see the negative possibilities in something new. That allows you to see that things 'going wrong' doesn't mean some kind of catastrophe, but may simply mean a different opportunity, a different experience.

Let me take you back to the example I gave above, when I used to attempt the 'double double' as part of my floor routine and I felt some fear around doing it. The odds of me experiencing negative physical consequences of getting it wrong were, in reality, low. I had practised it hundreds or even thousands of times, so if I got it wrong, it wouldn't be *that* wrong. I trusted that I knew what I was doing so I didn't really think I would hurt myself. My greater fear was around messing it up because it was such a difficult skill to perform, and therefore ruining my chances within the competition. So I had to flip the fear on its head and say to myself that whatever happens from this will be good for me. If I do it brilliantly then I will gain confidence and have a great chance in the competition. And if I mess it up then it will show me that I need to practise it more and, as a result, there will be another competition for me later down the line which I'll excel in.

With this perspective, there is nothing to fear about the uncertainty. Suddenly, I've removed any victim mentality that I might have over whether things will go as I expect them to. Instead, I've embraced the uncertainty as something that is perfectly normal and healthy. With this mentality, the crippling feeling that fear can give you can be replaced by the excited feeling that fear can give you.

There is a crucial element to all this – the victim mentality. I actually don't love that phrase because sometimes it is used to shame people, which isn't right. There are genuinely times when people are victims of bad things that have happened in life and they deserve every bit of sympathy. But there is a context in which it is used which I think is really important to understand, and it relates to feeling afraid about trying something new. If things don't go as we hope then one of the most unhelpful phrases we can tell ourselves is 'Why me?' – as in, 'What did I do to deserve this poor result? It's so unfair.' That mentality can seriously stop someone in their tracks in terms of moving forward in life.

I could have used it when I didn't feel the judges scored me highly enough in a competition or when someone cut me up on the road. You could use it if someone gets the promotion at work that you wanted or the tickets for the concert that you wanted to go to. The 'why me?' mentality firmly places you as a victim of consequences, as if it is in some way unfair on you. But that is essentially trying to make a deal with life that all uncertain aspects of it must fall how you want them to otherwise it is unfair! It's ridiculous really, but it is an easy mentality to slip into.

It's exactly what I talked about in the earlier chapter 'Why Me?' By adopting this mentality with every result that doesn't go your way, you are very unlikely to view something new or difficult with optimism. Your mentality is already halfway there to expecting a bad result that you can feel is unjust on you. Slipping into this mindset can be a comfortable position for some people, as it gives them a get-out before trying – 'Why bother if the result is very likely to be unfair on me!'

Once we flip our view on the uncertainties of life, we start to realise that life isn't doing anything *to* us, it is doing things *for* us. Of course, difficult things have happened and are going to happen to all of us, and everyone is allowed to feel sad, hurt or disappointed when they do. But that doesn't need to be the end point of how we view those outcomes in life. Life isn't doing unfair things *to* us; we are just temporarily experiencing difficult outcomes, which are part of a normal and uncertain life. Crucially, these hard, unwelcome results are going to lead us to greater growth – so much so that we might just look back on them with real gratitude one day, especially if we learn the lessons that they have the power to teach us.

If we can embrace this then we can even start to celebrate the uncertainty of life. We can stop fearing it and view all possibilities with abundance rather than limitation. Having an abundance mindset means viewing life positively, with great opportunities ahead of you, rather than negatively, in fear of terrible events to come. And remember, we have only talked about *if* the result doesn't go to plan. What if the plan goes far better than ever expected? This is a possibility that we have to remind ourselves at times. I used to enter every gymnastics competition with the intention of performing perfect routines on every apparatus, but that was never going to happen in reality. I'm human and we all make mistakes, so it's unrealistic to go through a series of skills or tests and expect nothing to go wrong. How I handled those mistakes in the middle of a competition was crucial, because fear could once again grip me for all the wrong reasons.

After a mistake, thoughts such as 'Oh no, this could be a terrible day' can come into your mind. That's pretty normal but you don't have to attach to it. You can have that thought but let it pass. Yes, it could be a terrible day, but it could also be an absolutely incredible day after that mistake. I could just be about to spark into life and perform some of the greatest routines that I have ever done in my life. Uncertainty doesn't always have to be about dealing with a poor result; it could be about anticipating an incredible result.

Let me give you an example of when I went to the 2014 European Junior Championships in Sofia, Bulgaria. I was 18, the captain and senior member of the team, and was expected to do very well. To be honest, there was a lot of pressure on me to perform. I qualified in first for the all-around final and was favourite to win. My first piece in the final was the vault, in which I performed reasonably. My next piece was the parallel bars, one of my strongest apparatuses, and I sat on the bar during a move called the Tippelt. That cost me a mark and meant I was lying in thirteenth place after the second rotation. To some people, that could have been disastrous and the end of their competition as they crumbled mentally, but, to this day, I clearly remember telling myself that I was still going to win. My attitude was that I could smash all of my next routines, take gold and have an incredible day. I didn't treat what was ahead of me with fear; instead I looked forward to the challenge. In the end, I did win gold after following up the mistake with four of my best routines as a junior gymnast on the next four pieces. It was a massive moment in my gymnastics career.

So, I want you to feel afraid at times in your life because it means you are pushing boundaries in order to help you grow as a person – we all need it. Understanding that fear and how to channel it is the crucial thing. Hopefully by now you can see that there is a way that you can feel excited about that fear rather than suffocated. It isn't an easy mentality to adopt and it will take practice, especially if this isn't a way that you have thought for a large part of your life. You will be essentially retraining your brain. If you feel yourself slipping into the victim mentality then pause yourself and start that thought process again. To begin with, there might be many times that you have to correct yourself, and that's OK. The more you do it, the more it will become you. You can reach a point in your life where, like me, you begin to search out challenges that will frighten you a little because they also excite you, and you know that whatever happens from it, you will grow as a person.

I hope you feel motivated to give it a go and develop this all-important mindset. While this chapter has explained how you can transform a powerful emotion like fear for your benefit, this next chapter is going to build on this to show you how you can face very difficult situations in a manner that can transform you from a state of unease to calmness.

FALLING OUT WITH PEOPLE

I have really struggled to deal with conflict throughout my life and it has a direct impact on my mental health. I don't know if it's because I'm a sensitive person, or it comes from an insecurity that means I always want to be liked, or that I just don't like seeing anyone upset – maybe it's a bit of all these things. But it is real – I'm not great in these situations. I don't feel at ease with conflict or difficulties in my relationships, and it can affect my confidence, self-esteem and my sleep.

Maybe you're like this too and spend a lot of your time trying to avoid conflict? Unfortunately, the reality is that conflict is part of life and it's important that we learn how to navigate it in a healthy way if we want to protect our mental health. I'm going to share with you how I have done this and I hope you can identify with it.

Last year, I broke up from a fairly long-term relationship and it was horrible. It wasn't the worst break-up of all-time but, still, I find these situations incredibly hard. They shine a light on some of the weaknesses I have with my mental wellbeing. I struggle with the thought of someone thinking badly of me and, all of a sudden, I'm alone with my thoughts and emotions, struggling with the noise in my own head. Which, as I've explained, is a real challenge for me.

Conflict can come along in lots of different ways, from an argument with someone close to you to a stranger being rude to you as you go through a door. When you are faced with some kind of conflict, you can feel an immediate rush of emotion that is unsettling. You might think this sounds strange coming from an athlete who is used to fronting up to difficult situations, but that is about competition, whereas this is about direct conflict. In the chapter 'Why We Keep Fucking Up', I gave you the example of when I publicly spoke out in the media about the culture within British gymnastics. I knew it was the right thing to do but it had a serious impact on my mental health. I couldn't cope with the fall-out from it as my mind raced, wondering if people hated me for doing it. What I have learned since then is that if I truly want to protect my mental health then I have to properly deal with conflict. Trying to avoid it or dodging the fact that I don't deal with these situations that well was never going to solve anything long-term.

Be honest

My first step in learning a better way to handle conflict was being brutally honest with myself. I had to accept that conflict has the potential to seriously knock me off the rails. This might sound really simple to you, and I guess it is, but that honesty wasn't always an easy thing for me to find. My ego got in the way of me accepting that I was very fragile in these situations. I didn't want to admit to anyone or even myself that if I broke up with my girlfriend, whether I wanted it or not, I would be extremely vulnerable and need help. And, as we've explored earlier, it can be difficult to ask for help. I think that women can be better at helping each other in these situations by talking it through with a friend, whereas men can end up getting quite isolated with it. I discovered that by letting go of that and accepting my vulnerability in this part of my life, I took a big step towards finding solutions.

Is this something you can relate to?

Has there been a challenge in your life that you got much closer to solving once you accepted that it was a vulnerability?

I'm sure you have noticed by now that a major theme of so much of what we have been talking about in these pages is a need for honesty and taking responsibility. We have to face up to this before we can move forward in almost anything. And it can be hugely liberating when we do. This is another great example.

De-centre yourself

The second step in this learning process for me was to understand that conflict is not all about me. This was a huge lightbulb moment because up to that point in time I didn't realise how self-obsessed I was in moments of conflict. I didn't do it with malice, but my focus in those situations was all about my own thoughts and emotions. I would just presume that someone's angry reaction to one of my actions was because they didn't like me anymore. Maybe they even hated me now. I basically took it as personally as you possibly could – it was all about me. I didn't take a moment to consider what was going on for the other person in the situation. Maybe they were having a really shit day. Maybe the way I had said something to them triggered a nerve in them from a way they had been treated in the past. Maybe they were feeling pressure in some other area in their life that I was completely unaware of and it was affecting their reaction. Maybe they had just received some really difficult news.

There are numerous other scenarios that could come into play with this. Have you had situations like this in which you have had an argument with someone and then later found out that there was something else that affected the whole disagreement, which was entirely separate to you?

I have learned that conflict doesn't *just* need to be centred on me and how I am feeling. It feels like a really obvious

FALLING OUT WITH PEOPLE

point as I write it, but it is just another one of those things that I've found difficult to appreciate. It reminds me of how isolating mental-health challenges can be. They narrow your world so much that you become hyperfocused on yourself. It's not through any bad intentions of selfishness, it's simply what's created in your mind. You find it really difficult to have an awareness beyond yourself.

The key to learning how to handle conflict better was to stop taking everything so personally, as if every argument or break-up was an intense reflection on my character. Once I began to grasp this, it actually felt like a relief. It felt like a burden was lifted from my shoulders. In the chapter 'What Holds Me Up in This World', I talk about how appreciating spirituality involves gaining an understanding that you are not in control of everything in the world. The same principle applies in dealing with conflict. During an argument, we can feel that we are directly in control of what someone thinks about us.

Learn to let go

Have you ever been trapped in an argument when you just want the other person to understand that you are 'right'? I definitely have. You end up going around in circles, and the end result is almost never that everyone blindly accepts that you were correct all along. If you have that mindset that you must 'prove' something to end the disagreement then the fall-out from it is going to greatly affect you because you are holding onto this illusion that you can control what some-one thinks about you. The alternative is to let go of needing to feel 'right'. You let go of wondering what the other person thinks about you. You even let go of what will happen next. And you are able to do this because you appreciate what you can and can't control. Where does the argument go from here? Nowhere. An argument requires two or more people to engage in it, and you have let go of it.

Shift your focus

I believe that we have all had that feeling when you can't sleep at night because you are still wrestling with an argu-ment in your head. Take yourself back to those sorts of moments and try to remember what would dominate your thoughts. If you are like me then it will be the other person. You'll be going over what they said, what they didn't under-stand, how they annoyed you, why they were wrong, what you think of them, and wondering what they think of you. Everything will be focused on them. This is a mental trap because there is no easy solution to it. You are ruminating about the other person while not being able to control them. All that will happen is that you'll continue to wrestle around with it in your mind because you want to make the other person believe, say and behave in exactly the way you want them to. This is not good for us because it not only disturbs our sleep, but it means we are focused on negativity. The antidote to this is, instead of focusing on what the other person was or wasn't saying, to focus entirely on yourself.

I would like you to think about a recent argument or disagreement you had with someone else. Ask yourself these questions:

1. Did you conduct yourself in a manner that you're proud of?
2. Did you put across your point of view as clearly as you could?
3. Did you keep your temper and avoid saying anything you regret?
4. Did you genuinely listen to the other person's opinions and feelings?

These questions are what you need to focus on to move past the negative aspects of that disagreement, not the other person. If the answer is 'yes' to all of these then you can be at ease knowing that you have done everything you could have done, and how the other person reacts is entirely up to them. If the answer is 'no' to one or more of those questions then you can quickly correct it. This might involve you meeting with the person again, but you will only be focused on correcting what you got wrong the first time, not reigniting the argument. Take responsibility for yourself and let everything else go. The phrase that I always use to remind myself of this is 'keep your side of the road clean'.

Keep your boundaries

I have learned that understanding boundaries so you can attempt to live in a solution rather than a problem is also key to helping me navigate conflict. Can you remember an argument you have had when things got out of hand and words were said that actually had no relevance to what the disagreement was about? If that's happened to you, like it has to me, then I suspect that the 'extra' things that were said were hurtful. When this happens the discussion often gets derailed badly and you get further away from a resolution. Being aware of boundaries within a disagreement is vital in being able to prevent this happening. Obviously, you can't prevent someone else from overstepping a boundary and saying something unnecessary and/or hurtful, but you can neutralise that by not engaging in it. Having an acute awareness of the boundary of the discussion means that you will only ever stick to what is relevant and helpful.

Do you have a memory of yourself or another person saying something like, 'Oh yeah, and while we're here', before unleashing a tirade about something completely separate to the argument? The times when this is at its most intense are when there is a lot of emotion involved, such as in a relationship break-up. Essentially, we verbally lash out because we are hurt, but when those things have been said, there is no taking them back. The harm can already be inflicted before we realise that we shouldn't have said it. If you can stay away from this then you are keeping the conversation in a place that's more likely to create a resolution.

Don't hold on to resentment

The last thing that I want to share with you is how to deal with things if you feel some residual resentment after an argument. Maybe you were hurt by something someone said or maybe you didn't feel they listened or respected you, and you can't let it go.

Take yourself back now to an argument that made you feel this way afterwards, and remind yourself of those emotions. In reality, it's common to feel like that – many people do after heated arguments. But holding onto that feeling isn't good for our mental health. It makes us feel unsettled and entrapped in negativity that drags us away from focusing on the daily actions that keep us healthy. You can be feeling all these horrible feelings towards someone and they can be blissfully unaware of it. It is a self-inflicted emotional pain that can stick in your head for far too long. It will affect your sleep, your concentration, your ability to stay present, your mood and your attitude. There is no positive from carrying around a resentment in your head.

There is a way to let go of this, but the size of the resentment will determine how much work you need to put into it. I always remind myself that if this is a resentment that has been left unresolved for years then I can't expect to unpick it in a matters of hours or even days. We can bury hurt a long way down in ourselves, and dealing with resentment involves bringing that back up to the surface, which isn't easy, fast or often that nice.

The fundamental way to resolve resentment is to empathise with the person who has caused you that hurt. I appreciate that this might be quite a difficult thing to hear if you have a long history with this person and you feel they have caused you a lot of harm. Nonetheless, practising empathy for them will release you from the self-inflicted burden of carrying a resentment.

I felt deeply hurt about a situation that arose with a member of staff at Leeds Gymnastics Club in December 2019. I reported it to British Gymnastics at the time, but my complaint was dismissed and it meant that I left what was my home club forever. I have spoken about it publicly. I felt so deeply hurt by it that the member of staff in question has lived in my thoughts for far too long. I'll admit that I hated that person for a period of time and I couldn't bear to hear their name. It felt so raw that I had to find a way to let it go. The only way I could do this was by developing empathy towards that person, which wasn't fucking easy! I could see that these actions must have come from somewhere, even if I could never know where, so I was able to develop a level of empathy for someone who found themselves in that emotional place in their life. It was so hard at times because every part of me wanted to continue hating them, but it was doing nothing for my mental health. It haunted me. So, every time I would get a negative thought about that person, I would stop myself and practise some empathy for them. I would remind myself that I didn't know everything about their life. As soon as I did this, the anger and bitterness behind my resentment would evaporate. The more I practised it, the more I would feel empathy rather than resentment. Even to this day, I have moments when my bitterness will flash back towards that person, but I immediately correct my thoughts and then quickly let go of the resentment. As a result, I am so much healthier.

I want you to take some time now to think back to one argument you have had and can remember clearly. Think through how it played out, what was said, how you behaved, how you felt afterwards and whether it became a long-running issue. Now think through all the steps I have described above and consider how you could have integrated them into what happened. Don't focus on whether it would have resolved the disagreement, because that's not entirely in your control, but instead think about whether it would have made a difference to how you felt afterwards.

Unfortunately, conflicts in life are unavoidable, whether big or small, but what we can control is how we react to them. A better understanding of all this is going to seriously help you with your mental health when faced with these difficult situations. You can remain far more stable rather than being thrown into a state of unease.

In the next chapter, I have thought about what I would tell my younger self having learned many of the lessons I have described so far. Before you take yourself there, take a moment to consider what you would tell your younger self. What is the most important lesson you feel you have learned about yourself or life, and how has this affected your mental health?

LIFE ISN'T HAPPENING TO YOU, IT'S JUST HAPPENING

If there was one thing that I could tell my younger self then it would be: 'nothing in life is permanent'.

Our thoughts, our emotions, our reactions and, there-fore, actions, change all the time. We've already talked a bit about the natural uncertainty there is to life. I have learned to embrace that in its many forms to maintain my mental wellbeing. So let's look at that in more detail here, as I want to challenge you to look at your own relationship with uncertainty in life and how it is affecting your mental health.

I have had, and still enjoy, some enormous highs in my life – the Olympics being the peak. I've also had some huge lows. As I look back on it all, I can see how many times in my life I have held onto a belief that whatever I was feeling at the time could well last forever – both good and bad. The highs I felt after the Rio Olympics were so powerful that I couldn't see how life would ever go back to normal.

And, likewise, the lows of my depression felt so bad that I never believed I would be able to get out of that hole. But the end of the story, on both fronts, is that those feelings didn't last forever, however powerful they were at the time.

By nature, I think I am someone who is always going to be susceptible to big highs and lows in my life – and maybe you are the same. It's part of who I am because I shoot for the stars and, as I have mentioned before, I am also very sensitive. It's something that I've learned to understand about myself and have become much better at managing. For a long time, though, I just thought it was how life was for me – which reflected my lack of self-awareness then. I have found that once that switch is turned on to appreciate self-awareness, it never goes, but, before that, you have no idea that you lack it.

Looking back, my attachment to highs and lows was dangerous. In 2018, I was one of the fastest-growing YouTubers in the UK. My total views, subscriber growth and engagement were off the charts. It was impossible not to get caught up in the hype and adrenaline of it all, it was fucking crazy! At the time, I didn't see any reason why this success wouldn't go on and on. I could just keep pumping out content and everyone would love it and me forever. Maybe I didn't give it that much thought, but I definitely never had a moment of true perspective on it all. I still financially benefit from YouTube very well, but that level of growth in 2018 was never going to continue at the same rate. It was impossible because nothing is permanent in life. People weren't going to love my content at the same level of intensity forever, and it was ridiculous to expect that. People's preferences change all the time – I mean, which comedy show or singer has been at the top of the top forever? None. I didn't know it, but that level of success was always going to be temporary for me because *everything* is. I didn't need to take the whole experience personally, and I mean that in both ways – the success wasn't because I was a superhuman and the eventual slowdown of it all wasn't because I was a failure. It hit me hard when my level of success started to change, and this was all because I didn't have any real perspective on the transient nature of all things in life.

Maybe you have had moments like this in your life too when success at work or in another part of your life seems to come really easily and then suddenly disappear. Maybe you had achieved consecutive yearly promotions at work then it stopped without you realising why. Maybe you had a really happy friendship group and then everyone started falling out.

Take a moment to consider if this sort of thing has happened in your own life.

How did this change make you feel?

Exactly the same dynamic existed when I was crippled with depression and anxiety. I remember one particular night when I was in bed with a past girlfriend. Everything was good at that moment in time. We were cuddling and she was falling asleep. I finished watching some snooker on my phone, put my head on the pillow and then bang! it was there. Anxiety just engulfed me. I started crying. My girl-friend woke up and asked me what was wrong. All I could say was, 'I don't fucking know.' I was shaking, heavy breath-ing and crying. I had to go and sit outside on my balcony, and I couldn't sleep until 4am.

I spent all that night and the following days wondering what the hell was wrong with me. I thought I'd changed and become this incredibly fragile person. An Olympian had become a crying wreck. It was such a crippling and over-whelming experience that I couldn't see how things would return to how they were previously. In the confusion of it all, I wondered if I had changed forever. It was all so real that it was hard not to think that. I couldn't grasp any real perspective on it in exactly the same way I didn't with my crazy YouTube success in 2018. Even though the emotions in each situation were polar opposites, I didn't realise how much I expected them to stay like that and the impact that would have on me. I have since learned that everything passes eventually – like clouds in the sky.

I can now see the understanding that nothing is perman-ent in life is a perspective or an attitude that eventually just becomes part of who you are. I can see it in other people who seem to move with the flow of life so effortlessly. They don't get too carried away when everything is perfect, nor do they get too down when things are not so good. More than anything, they don't take life personally – life isn't happening to them, it's just happening.

I actually used to be quite suspicious of these sorts of people – I would be like, 'Do they not care enough about things?' and, 'Are they faking this?' I found it quite a difficult mindset to get my head around. I have since realised that it was because I was so attached to the huge highs and the huge lows in life that I couldn't imagine that there was another way to live. I guess I also worried that anything other than extremes would be quite boring, grey, vanilla, and I didn't want that. I believed that I would rather have the rollercoaster of life than anything too 'medium'.

But I have discovered that living in a flow with life isn't grey or boring – quite the opposite, in fact. Having an appreciation that everything is transient doesn't mean that you can't absolutely love the wonderful things that come into your life. Winning *Dancing on Ice* was a massive buzz for me and I loved it all! I loved the acclaim, the achievement, the fun and most definitely the celebration – I loved it all to the max. But the difference with that and what happened when I came back from the Olympics in 2016 was that I fundamentally knew that life would return to normal when it all subsided – and that was totally fine with me.

I guess all of this ties into what I was talking about earlier in terms of spirituality – my trust in the universe to sort all the outcomes as they are meant to be while I keep doing the next right thing (flip back to 'Every Damn Day' for a reminder). I'm not a religious person in the slightest and don't really have any concept of god, but I have begun to see how an appreciation of life being bigger than just what I think and presume is really healthy. To see that things naturally change in life is, to me, to understand that the world is moving around me whether I like it or not. And, do you know what? When I started to have this shift in my mindset, it was a fucking relief on so many levels!

Firstly, not everything was on me. I realised that I didn't need to carry the weight of always being successful at everything because it wasn't *all* on me – I just needed to always put my best foot forward. And secondly, it made me see during difficult times with my mental health or other things in life that the bad times wouldn't last forever – they would pass.

During dark times, when I have wanted to escape the mental pain I was in through alcohol or gambling or whatever else, it was because I couldn't cope with the moment. A big part of that was because I didn't appreciate that it would eventually pass. I couldn't see any light at the end of the tunnel and I felt suffocated. But now I have this appreciation that there is always something else coming down the road, even if you can't see it yet. There is always light at the end of the tunnel.

It's a silly example, but this point always reminds me about the story as to why Uber brought in a tracking map for you to see where your car was and how long it would take to get to you. The map has never made cars get to people quicker – availability and traffic obviously dominate that – but Uber realised that the thing that upset customers the most was not the actual wait, it was not knowing how long the wait would be. Once they introduced the map, people were much calmer about the wait.

It's not dissimilar to when I used to do some excruciating exercises during my early years in gymnastics to increase my flexibility. To improve our splits, we used to have our feet over two blocks and be suspended in the middle off the ground. Our legs would be beyond horizontal in an over split. It was so painful it would bring me to tears. We would even hang 5kg weights off each foot to make it harder. It was unbearable, but there was a key factor it – it would last one minute. As bad as it was, I knew that it would be over after 60 seconds. Suffering is horrible, but knowing that it will come to an end at some point makes it so much easier to cope with.

Spirituality can be a big concept to get our heads around and sometimes triggers strong reactions. How does it feel for you reading what I've said about it? At times people connect it to religion. They then react based on what their views are on religion. I used to do the same. But I've learned that it isn't about that – it's not about believing or not believing in a god or gods. This is about having an appreciation of a universe beyond ourselves and, therefore, understanding what is and isn't in our control.

Maybe like you, I found this a tough idea to embrace to start with. The reason being that I didn't like believing that I wasn't in control of everything. I liked the idea that I could make anything happen if I worked hard enough at it. Believing in anything bigger than me was at odds with this.

I'd like you to take some time now to consider these concepts. Ask yourself: how much of what may or may not happen in your life do you believe is in your control? If you think you control all or most of it then think about how much pressure that puts on you. This might be the first time you have ever considered this so take your time with it and write your thoughts down. When you've finished doing this, ask yourself how you think it would feel if you allowed yourself to let go of some of that pressure by accepting that you're not in total control of all outcomes in your life?

Don't rush this process. It might help you to think of situations that you got yourself wrapped up in a mental knot over. Particularly think of situations that had a detrimental effect on your mental health. Maybe it was after a job interview or wanting something to happen at work? Maybe it involved a relationship you're in or when you have tried to help a friend with a difficult situation? These are situations that have played on your mind day and night. You probably tried to stop thinking about them but they dominated you for a period of time.

Take yourself back to there and analyse how much you ruminated over it. Maybe you couldn't stop thinking about whether you had done everything correctly in the situation and how that would affect the outcome. Now imagine that in one of those situations someone had told you that you had done everything perfectly because you had tried your best and the result was out of your control. How would it feel to let go of the responsibility for the outcome because you simply did your best?

I believe that if you can do this, you will feel one over-riding emotion – relief. It is that exact feeling that is the start of embracing spirituality. Keep exploring this.

I want you all to shoot for the stars in life. Challenge yourself as much as possible because it is a win-win. You will grow from every experience and I believe that is truly living life. Be ambitious and daring, celebrate your successes and learn quickly when things don't go to plan, and hang in there when things are really tough. Knowing that everything will pass, both the good and the bad, shouldn't deter you from this sort of mindset in the slightest. A broader appreciation of the journey of life just allows you to find a stability that you can enjoy and enables you to cope with everything better. All of this is absolutely vital for looking after your mental health.

In this next chapter, I want to continue the theme of how we view life and how it affects our mental health. A simple change of perspective can be truly transformational, and I'm excited to share this next one with you.

LIVE IN THE NOW

I want you to take a moment now to think back on a day when everything was, well, a bit shit. A day when nothing seemed to happen as you would have liked it to and everything felt difficult. Maybe it was a day during this last week or even today? You know, one of those days when you ended up having a needless argument or you got upset over something relatively minor. Your gratitude for life would not have been an all-time high on a day like this. But here's the magic – that crappy day only lasts for 24 hours. When you finally get yourself to bed at the end of that day, it's over. You wake up the next day and you can start all over again.

We don't know with any real certainty what is going to happen in the next 24 hours, so every day, life essentially gives us another shot at it and I fucking love that! We have been given this beautiful opportunity to experience what it's like to be a human being, but it is broken down into one day at a time. However shit your day before has been, you can immediately put it behind you and start again.

Appreciating this has helped me so much with my mental health because it has enabled me to remain far more present in life. What I mean by 'present' is that rather than getting caught in thoughts or worries about the past or the future, I can just focus on the 24-hour cycle of life in front of me. Just one day at a time. This understanding has allowed me to move away from the trap set by anxiety that keeps your mind obsessively worried about the past and the future.

Have you ever looked at life this way? Have there been times when you have allowed one bad day to affect so many more in your week when it really didn't need to? Can you see how you can change this now?

I have talked a lot throughout this book about the compounding effect of decisions – good or bad – on how we manage our mental health, and I would like you to consider what I am explaining here within this context too. Each new day represents an opportunity for us to start again, and if something isn't working to stop doing it and try something else.

For example, in 2019, I was making bad decisions all the time, particularly with alcohol. My mental health was shot to pieces but I wasn't helping myself at all. Do you remember I told you about the time when I really let my sister down in the corporate hospitality at the cricket that she had arranged? I messed up badly that day, but what I can now see is that I let that continue into the following days. I didn't see the next day and the one after that as opportunities to be better; I could only see that I had messed up, was a waste of space and would continue to be one. So, my poor decisions continued. Looking back, I can see that I didn't need to do this.

Being able to stay present in life is a beautiful and important mindset to have. Without it, I could be trying to make a cup of tea and yet be consumed by paranoia over something that happened the day before. The action of making and then drinking the tea can feel like a version of autopilot while my mind is occupied with unhealthy trains of thought.

Do you relate to that? Are there times when you are trying to do things but your mind wants to fixate on things away from it? Have you found yourself unable to appreciate or enjoy anything in front of you? The taste of that cup of tea basically becomes irrelevant while your mind is trapped in anxious thoughts. Maybe you have felt this when spending time with your family or friends?

I don't have children, but I hear parents talk about how anxiety ruins their time with their kids, as they can't get themselves truly present. In those moments, life is just passing us by. Children are growing up while our minds are obsessed by things away from that beauty. The present moment basically becomes nothing more than background noise. I don't want to live my life like that and I suspect you don't either. We have this incredible opportunity of life and yet it can just drift by us.

The 24-hour cycle that I am talking about in this chapter is a perfect antidote to this. Imagine for a moment how it would feel to have one day left to live. What went before would have little or no importance and there would obviously be no future, you would just have that single day left. I think most of us have had that chat with a friend at some point in our lives, saying, 'What would you do if you had one day left to live?' Not everyone's answer would be the same, but there is one thing that would be – we would all want to cherish every single moment of that day. We would want to taste anything we ate or drank as richly as we could. We would want to powerfully feel every emotion. We would want to hear and say every word as clearly as possible. We would want to absorb absolutely everything from that day because it would be our last. That is being truly present. Take a moment now to consider how this fits into the mind-set of looking at life as a series of 24-hour opportunities.

If you can wake up seeing the day ahead of you as a brand now opportunity to experience the brilliance of life then what happened the day before is only a reference point. Yesterday will be full of learnings from both good and bad things that happened throughout the day, but that doesn't mean it will dictate what's next. If you can hold that mindset then it is extraordinarily powerful in making you present.

There is a strong connection here to the thoughts I have shared about spirituality. It all links to a mindset of letting go of what has happened and believing in something bigger to guide what's next for you. Compare this with what your mind does when you feel crippled by anxiety. If you're like me, then it will be the exact opposite. Your mind will be catastrophising about everything that has happened and may happen in your life. You feel like you should be able to control this but you simply don't have the ability to. It's horrible. What I am talking about here is a combination of letting go of what has been and trusting in what will come next.

Let's move this forward now to the end of the day when you climb into bed. If it's been a difficult day then maybe your mind is consumed by everything that's happened. Do you struggle to sleep in those situations? I have, many times. It comes from a lack of acceptance of what is. Now link this to what we are talking about in this chapter. As you climb into bed, you can mentally take note that the day has gone, it's over. You will learn from what's happened but tomorrow morning will signify a new day, a new opportunity for life. If you're able to do this – and it will take practice – you can truly adopt a liberating mindset of acceptance that will enormously benefit your mental health.

The more you do it, the more it will just become how you live your life, and you will need fewer mental reminders to yourself.

There is another place that you can take this mindset to help you even more with staying present. Can you view life as a series of 'nows' in which your day is a chain of events? This can be simple things like brushing your teeth, as well as bigger things like an important work meeting. Can you view them as individual events and treat them accordingly? For example, when you brush your teeth can you fully concentrate on the job in hand by focusing on each tooth and each brushstroke to do the best job you possibly can? When you're in your work meeting, can you be entirely engrossed with what's happening in the meeting without being distracted? When you meet up with a friend, are you listening to everything they are saying, or thinking about what has just happened or what you are doing next?

Consider again what you would do if it was your last day on earth. You would want to be entirely present for all these things. If you view each 'now' or event as the most important thing happening in your life at that moment, then you will stay completely present with it. You will be bringing the best version of yourself to whatever you are doing.

If you think this is going to be a struggle for you because you have such a racing mind then I want you to try something now. Take a moment to go outside or look out of the window. Look for the edges of building or of trees. Or even look for the gaps between branches or buildings. Try this for five minutes and then step away and reflect on how your mind was in those moments. It will have been entirely present with no other thoughts distracting you. Your mind would have been focused on those edges or those gaps. That is your proof as to how you can focus your mind. The challenge now is whether you can take this into the individual events that happen in your day. If you are finding this difficult in the course of a day then take a moment again to look for edges or gaps around things near you and it will bring your mind back in the moment.

I believe that if we can achieve this sort of present mind-set, then we are truly living because we are appreciating everything in front of us. We are pulling together everything I have talked about throughout this chapter and, rather than sleepwalking through life while preoccupied by the past and the future, we are arriving at each moment, giving it our whole attention. In doing this, we present the best version of ourselves to any given moment, and it is that version that helps us to maintain the best possible mental health.

WHAT NOW?

I want you to focus on where you go now with everything you've read in this book. It might feel like there is a lot to absorb and you need time to reflect back on some of topics that I have discussed. I appreciate that I have challenged you to be really honest with yourself, and that doesn't always come immediately or easily. But finding that honesty within yourself is vital for moving forward using the tools I have shown you.

It feels like so much has become about programmes to follow to improve something in our lives – whether it be our finances, our fitness, our diet and even our mental health. I understand this because people crave guidance and structure, so something in a formulated programme feels reassuring. But we have to be careful that some fundamental things aren't lost in all of this.

One is that we are all different – what works for one

person might not for another, and that is OK. We don't all like the same food, same workouts, same sports, same books, same films, etc, so why would the same 'improve yourself' set of instructions work for us all? Educating yourself as best you can through reading, listening and watching other people talk about it is a very important part of learning to manage your mental health, but it doesn't mean all of it will be exactly right for you. Try out the approaches you learn, keep an open mind, but don't feel you have to follow everything that someone else does. What I have found works for me is a combination of things I have learned from lots of different people and situations. I would never want you to read this book and see me as telling you exactly what it is you need or should do; instead, I hope that in sharing my experience and what works for me, I have given you an opportunity to take from it what you want. I believe that if we get into a 'tick box' exercise created by someone else then we might just be creating more problems for ourselves. If the programme that we have been told will work doesn't work, what the hell do we do then? That loneliness of mental-health issues returns but with even more vengeance.

Another important thing I think we need to be aware of is how so much can become dominated by comparison. Social media is a massive part of my life and, overall, I love it – but I can also see it for what it is. It breeds comparison! There was a period of time on Instagram when it felt like if you weren't having an ice bath every morning then you were virtually inviting depression and anxiety into your life! When an online environment is created in which people who are desperately looking for help get told what they *must* do rather than what they *could* do it can be so counterproductive. Vulnerable people will follow the advice but not necessarily for the right reasons.

If we become so focused on following what everyone else tells us is right for us and what everyone else is doing then we are naturally going to compare. Comparison has such a terrible effect on our mental health and it can invite loneliness – 'Well, that person is doing their ice baths and they look really happy, but I'm doing it and I still feel like shit.' Comparison gives too much space for people to believe they are 'failing', and that is never true. I have talked about the importance of community within the book, and allowing vulnerable people to feel like they are failing is not what a mental-health community should be all about. So, I urge everyone to help others by sharing your experience in a way that allows people to learn from it, rather than ramming it down someone's throat as if they must do it.

I want you to measure yourself on progression, not perfection, going forward. The idea that we can perfectly manage our mental health is an illusion that can sometimes suffocate us. If we're not getting it right and feeling good all the time then we can tell ourselves that we are failing. That's not true. This is just about forward movement – sometimes that's big leaps, and at other times it's tiny steps. Maybe you have even made progress as you have been reading this book, and that is fantastic.

Let progression be your only barometer going forward.

I, for one, can proudly tell you that I am a work in progress. It might even sound odd to you that I say I am 'proud' of this, but I really am. There is no such place as being 'recovered' from mental-health issues and, importantly, nor should there be. Before I explain why, it is worth pointing out that the concept of being fully on top of any sort of health issue is a really odd one. We don't ever tell people that we are completely on top of our physical health because the truth is that we don't know. People can do their best with their lifestyle and diet and still get ill seemingly from nowhere. We just do our best. The idea of fully recovering mental health is equally flawed. Going back to the point I made in the last chapter that life changes all the time, how can we ever really know if we will suffer from a bout of depression or anxiety again? We can't.

But there is a fundamental reason why I am proud of being a 'work in progress'. Understanding that I always need to do work in this area to take good care of myself and that I don't always have the answers keeps me grounded. It's a mindset that makes sure that through my humility I continually respect the challenges mental health can throw at me. Because if I get too big for my boots and believe that I am 'recovered' and know everything there is to know about it, then it comes around to bite me very fast!

I have found that learning to manage my mental health can be a very humbling experience. As you'll have seen, I now know what I need to do to give myself the best possible chance of maintaining a good handle on my mental health, but that all has to happen alongside a big chunk of humility.

I do feel in a fantastic place in my life now and am incredibly grateful for the lessons that I've learned, some of which have been really hard. I still chase incredible goals, particularly in business, but I move with the flow of life far better now by enjoying the journey of what I am doing rather than fixating on results. Most importantly, I have learned to surrender to life rather than resist it. Today, I submit to what's in front of me in life at any given time and then move to the solution. I don't resist or refuse to accept an outcome, whether I like it or not – and this really applies to my mental health too.

I can't say this strongly enough: finding a healthy way to manage your mental health is not about fighting, it is about surrendering. A 'fight' is still trapped in that thought that comes from ego, a belief that there will be a winner and a loser, as there is in every fight eventually. This mentality served me well as an athlete because I would fight everything, through pain, setbacks and obstacles. It was all I knew. But in managing my mental health, this hasn't served me. It's an illusion if we perceive that we are 'fighting' our mental-health challenges. If I hear someone say 'I am going to beat this thing' when they are referring to depression, anxiety or another mental-health issue, then I am concerned for them. This is about surrendering to what it is, accepting it and quickly moving into solutions.

As I've said, the same applies to life in general. Those nights that we toss and turn in bed, not being able to sleep because there is something bugging us about what happened in the day, happen because we are simply not accepting what is. We wrestle with whatever is bugging us because we don't want it to have happened and we can't let go of it. But, if we surrender to it then we accept it, and we have the opportunity to move to a solution. Like with everything in this book, it takes practice, and it might not come naturally to everyone, but take some time to consider this the next time you can't sleep because something is still annoying you from the day that just happened.

Maybe the most important thing I have realised about my life now is that I am in charge of myself. And I'm not saying that casually – I fucking mean that from the deepest part of my being. This is tightly linked to that honesty that I have challenged you to search for in your life. I needed to get brutally honest with myself to accept that what is and isn't in my life today is down to the responsibility I am taking for my life on a day-to-day basis.

Take a moment now to consider this again because it is *so* important. Do you feel you are being honest with yourself about the actions you take in your life? Do you feel in charge of yourself or do you feel simply at the will of things that happen to you? As you do this, remind yourself not to confuse responsibility with control. I definitely don't believe that I can control everything that happens in my life, but I am in charge of my reaction to every outcome within it. My mental health is absolutely included in that. There are times when my mental health takes a dive for reasons out of my control, but what I know is that I am in charge of what I do about that. I make choices on a daily basis to maintain the best mental health possible, and I make choices to help myself out of a hole when I am in it.

Being fully responsible for all the choices I make in my life means taking ownership of trying to be the best version of myself I can be and not expecting anyone else or anything else to do it for me. I have made mistakes and will make more, but that's because I am human. I am not my mistakes but I control what I do after I make mistakes. Today I am in charge of who I am and I fucking love that.

This mentality or attitude has given me a freedom in life that I never knew existed. Being in charge of myself isn't just about taking responsibility, it is also about knowing who I am and how I want to live my life. Hopefully, having read this book, you can now really see this about me. Having this certainty about who I want to be is a real liberation. I'm not trying to be anything to anyone else or trying to chase something about myself that I feel is missing. I finally feel that everything I might need in life is within me.

Just like everyone, especially when we're young, I have been self-conscious about my appearance, my status and what people think of me, but I have realised that comes with chains. You are chained to trying to be something or to fit in to what you think you're supposed to be rather than having a real handle on yourself. You end up living your life in a way that you think looks 'right' through the eyes of other people, which is an impossible trap on so many levels. You will never be able to fully satisfy that because you will become hypersensitive to different people's changing opinions. But, most importantly, you are very likely to end up living a life that bears little resemblance to who you are as a person. While you scamper around trying to make things look as you think they should for others, you will lose yourself. You will lose what your values are, what makes you happy, and, eventually, you will entirely lose who you are. So, that's why I say that being in charge of yourself is the great freedom in life. Whatever outcomes happen in my life, good and bad, I am in charge of who I am and the choices that I make.

My manager, Luke, often reminds me of this quote from an Ancient Greek Stoic philosopher called Epictetus: 'If your choices are beautiful, so too will you be.' Understanding how and why we make our choices in life has been an important underlying theme throughout this book. It's essentially what self-awareness is. I guess we could ask what makes a choice 'beautiful'. Well, for me it is pretty simple. Am I being of service to others? Am I using my abilities in the best way I can? Am I running towards something rather than away from something? If you too ask yourself these questions and the answer to all is 'yes' then feel assured that your choice is a good one, or a 'beautiful' one. It doesn't mean that you'll always make the best choice available, but you now have an ability to see this mistake and make a better one next up.

I'm so grateful that I got the opportunity to write this book. It has given me a chance to reflect on everything I have learned. I will read this book whenever I need it and there will definitely be times in the future when that will be the case. I really wish for you to use it in the same way. I suspect there will be chapters of this book that you connect with more than others, and that's OK. You can go back to just the bits that you want to remind yourself about whenever you like. If you feel you have lost your way in managing your mental health then please read it again, and don't forget the phrase I used earlier in this chapter – measure yourself on progression, not perfection. It truly is progression to come back to this book when you need it, even if you feel in a hole at the time. It's a version of asking for help, and it's important to acknowledge to yourself how positive that is for you.

This book also gave me another opportunity to be a voice for mental health and I love that. The loneliness that you feel when trapped by poor mental health is really horrible, and the more we talk about it, the less anyone has to feel alone when suffering from it.

I want this book to be for everyone, whatever age, gender or background you are. Though I also see that, as I am a young man, this book might resonate strongly with other men. If that's the case then there is something really important in that for me. The suicide rate for men is still so alarmingly high and, sadly, the conversation around mental health sometimes still hits a stumbling block with men. We don't talk about it anywhere near enough, especially with each other. I believe it's because of the trap of the old stereotype of what being a man is.

Our fathers are from a generation taught to believe that men always need to be strong and not show vulnerability. For their fathers, this was even more intense. Things have softened over generations and it has got better, but it's not fixed. My generation represents change with regards to men talking about their issues, but there is still a lot of work left to do. That old construct of a man can often stop us from letting go and allowing ourselves to be vulnerable in front of others, especially other men. Chatting about football in the pub can be much easier for us than chatting about our feelings, which can leave a lot of men trapped inside their heads, believing that they need to sort their problems on their own. It blows my mind that men can sometimes only show real emotion when their team score a goal or they have had a few beers – it shouldn't be that way. Telling our 'other halves' is a possible outlet, but that trap of feeling that we always need to appear strong can often hold us back again. I believe that all men want to feel like a strong person within a family unit; I honestly think it is something primal. However, we need to let go of the mistaken belief that discussing our feelings and showing vulnerability is somehow a weakness. It is not. It is a strength. There is so much more that needs to be done in this area and that's why I love having a platform to talk about it. How we talk about it is crucial, though.

I hope you have gained some important perspective and tools from this book. If it is the first time you have ever read a book like this then the realisation that you are not alone with your mental-health challenges may have made a difference to you. I have had the same extremely difficult and confusing thoughts and feelings you have. We are all part of a community that can help each other, so please tell people around you what you have learned from this book. The more knowledge people have, the more solutions we will have to help.

I will continue talking about mental-health issues and what we can do about them as far and widely as I can. Please engage with me on social media and share with me your opinions on managing your mental health. I really do welcome all comments that you have. If we are to keep the conversation around mental health moving forward then the more engagement the better. Tell me what works for you, what doesn't work for you and how it all feels.

Let's keep talking and helping each other.

ACKNOWLEDGEMENTS

Luke Sutton – You saved my life, thank you for standing by me, educating me and speaking my language when I needed it most.

Mum, Dad, Joanna – Sorry for putting you through hell at times, although it wouldn't be the Wilson way without it. I love you more.

ABOUT THE AUTHOR

Nile Wilson is one of Great Britain's greatest ever gymnasts and has been a trailblazer for the sport in many different ways. He won a bronze medal in the horizontal bar at the 2016 Rio Olympics, which was Team GB's first ever Olympic medal in the discipline. Yet, Nile is so much more than just a gymnast – a YouTuber with over 1.5 million subscribers and 350 million total views; a social-media influencer; a highly successful entrepreneur; an advocate for mental-health awareness; and a powerful voice within his sport over the historic treatment of gymnasts.

Nile has also been brutally honest about the battles he has faced with his own mental health. After a serious neck injury in 2019, Nile's world began to fall apart as he became swamped with depression, anxiety and addictive behaviours. His documentary *The Silent Battle*, in which he and his family gave incredible insight into what happened during this period of time and how he rose from it, has been watched by more than a million people. Nile's honesty on this subject has been incredibly rare not only for an athlete of his profile, but also, importantly, a male one.

In March 2023, Nile was crowned champion of ITV's *Dancing on Ice* in front of a TV audience of nearly 5 million people. During this period of time, Nile gained some real clarity on what helps him and, maybe even more crucially, what doesn't help him in maintaining stability with his mental health. Nile is now ready to share all of these crucial lessons in this book.

Follow Nile on Instagram (@nilemw), YouTube (@NileWilsonGymnast), TikTok (nilewilsonator) and Facebook (NileWilsonGymnast).